Ian
Frazer

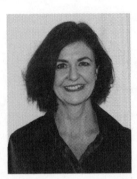

Madonna King is an award-winning journalist, commentator and author. She has spent 25 years working as a journalist in Brisbane, Sydney, the Canberra press gallery and the United States.

This is Madonna's fourth book. Her previous titles include *Catalyst*, which looks at the media, politics and the law; *One-Way Ticket* (co-authored with Cindy Wockner), an investigation into the lives of the Bali 9; and *A Generous Helping* (co-authored with Alison Alexander), which drew on the community to create a best-selling recipe collection to raise money for victims of the 2011 Queensland floods.

Madonna also writes a weekly column for *The Courier-Mail*, sits on three not-for-profit boards, and travels Australia facilitating and moderating events. She is married to David, and they have two daughters.

For more information, see www.madonnaking.com.au

Ian Frazer

MADONNA KING

First published 2013 by University of Queensland Press
PO Box 6042, St Lucia, Queensland 4067 Australia

www.uqp.com.au
uqp@uqp.uq.edu.au

Cover design by Nada Backovic
Cover photograph by Justine Walpole
Typeset in 11.5/16 pt bembo by Post Pre-press Group, Brisbane
Printed in Australia by McPherson's Printing Group
All photographs supplied by the Frazer family unless otherwise stated.

National Library of Australia Cataloguing-in-Publication data
is available at http://catalogue.nla.gov.au/

Ian Frazer: The man who saved a million lives / Madonna King
ISBN (hbk) 978 0 7022 5002 6
ISBN (pbk) 978 0 7022 4957 0
ISBN (pdf) 978 0 7022 5183 2
ISBN (epub) 978 0 7022 5184 9
ISBN (kindle) 978 0 7022 5185 6

University of Queensland Press uses papers that are natural, renewable and recyclable
products made from wood grown in sustainable forests. The logging and manufacturing
processes conform to the environmental regulations of the country of origin.

To my daughters Madison and Siena. Never stop trying.
This story explains why.

JACINTA STEWART couldn't escape work so was late when she tiptoed in halfway through the speech being delivered in the Monash Room at the Australian Consulate in New York. She sat down quietly, surveying the audience who were listening intently to the guest speaker, and waited for the opportunity to jump to her feet. Her best chance to make herself known this June day had been the coffee break, but it had been cancelled to make up time after guests watched Australia playing Italy in the FIFA World Cup. Now Ian Frazer, the recently minted Australian of the Year, had finished his speech and was answering research and science questions posed by the audience.

The session was winding up. It was now or never, Jacinta thought. She began to raise her arm tentatively, and then threw it up in the air, determined to be heard. Most questions had related to Ian Frazer's medical research, and the need for government funding; her interest in both of these areas was limited. She had another reason for being in this room on this day, and had RSVPed to the meet-and-greet the moment she saw it pop up in her email. The facilitator beckoned towards her, asking her to stand. And then Jacinta Stewart patted down her white denim jacket and turned to the man who was receiving accolades the world over for stopping the virus that causes cervical cancer; the man whose determination over the previous fifteen years would end up saving the lives of 275,000 women who would otherwise die of the disease each year; the man who Jacinta Stewart had not seen since she lay in a hospital bed fearing for her life.

'I would like to propose a toast,' she said, grabbing an empty wine glass off the person sitting next to her, 'for something you did seventeen years ago.' She was on a roll now. She had wanted to do this for so long, and now she had Ian Frazer's attention. He was looking at her, listening to every word she spoke. 'You made a diagnosis that saved my life. I was admitted to the Mater hospital in Brisbane in a life-threatening stage. You visited me as a special favour and I never got to thank you.'

Ian Frazer didn't take his eyes off her, but took over the conversation. Who was the physician, he asked. When was it? And then the penny dropped. 'I remember,' he said. 'You were very sick. It was Christmas Eve. Your family was so upset.'

For the second time, Jacinta was struck by the bedside manner of the man she believed had saved her life. How could he remember that fleeting moment seventeen years ago that had given her a second chance at life? She started to cry. For years, in fact at every significant milestone after her illness, her father had rallied the family, raised a glass and said, 'Thank God for Ian Frazer.' Now that her father had passed away, it was her turn. She raised her glass. 'Thank God for Ian Frazer,' she said.

The two people sitting next to Jacinta burst into tears too. The audience hung on every word, looking between the young woman who was on her feet, and the guest of honour. Professor

Ian Frazer, the Scottish-born medico who rose through the science labs to become one of Australia's best imports, looked back at her in the sea of faces. He was used to being feted by the rich and famous. He had taken out almost every science prize on offer for the co-discovery that led to the first vaccine that could stop cancer. Looking outside the window, where you could see both the Empire State Building and the Chrysler Building, New York was in its daily overdrive. Taxis whizzed by, New Yorkers rushed between cars. People ate their lunch on the run. The subway labyrinth pulled people in at some stops and spat them out at others. But inside this room it was silent. Jacinta held her breath and waited for Ian Frazer to answer her. She willed him to say something, but she didn't quite know what.

'I would like to say something,' he said slowly and deliberately. 'Thank you, Jacinta, for reminding me in this moment of why I do what I do.'

One

Marion Frazer first remembers the piercing blue eyes. Her son, Ian Hector Frazer, had only just been born and placed in a crib by her side. She looked at him, and he stared back with eyes a shade of blue she had never seen before. It was Tuesday 6 January 1953, and she and her husband, Sam, wondered what life would hold for their firstborn.

Their union had been a whirlwind romance. Sam had a medical degree, was studying biochemistry and held a position as a junior lecturer at Glasgow University when he offered fellow lecturer and science graduate Marion Shepherd a lift to work. The city of Glasgow, which had been an engine room for industry at the close of the Second World War, now found itself facing decline as the economies of Europe revived. Smog clung to the city's buildings, stripping colour from the sky. Over a cup of coffee, Sam Frazer and Marion Shepherd talked, fell in love, and married nine months later in St Andrew's Chapel. Eleven months later, on a near-freezing winter's day, Ian arrived.

It wasn't long before independence characterised his young personality. Before he could crawl, Marion remembers him rolling over and over to reach for what he wanted. He was determined, persistent, and never screamed for assistance. But he almost always got his own way, and by the time his sister, Lesley, was born in November the following year, that spark of independence really shone. Even when he could talk, Ian preferred to work things out by himself, shunning help from those years older, and that's what his playmates first noticed when the family followed Sam from Glasgow to a senior lecturership at The University of Edinburgh.

The young family stayed in rented accommodation in Edinburgh first, before moving to Braid Hills in the city's south-west. Two more children arrived in quick succession: Neil in January 1956, and Ewan in November 1958, and a nanny joined them too, to help Marion with their four young children.

Young Gerrard Clark lived next door. A big vacant lot lay between 12 and 16 Braid Mount, but a house was soon built on it, and, when the new family moved in, he clambered over the fence to meet them. The house was big, with a bedroom for each child. At number 16 Braid Mount, Keith Maclennan also watched, hoping the tall young boy called Ian would become his new friend too.

It wasn't long before the three boys – Ian, Gerrard and Keith – became pals. The Braid Hills area overflowed with families, and almost all the children attended the local Merchant Company school, George Watson's College. They were part of a community that laid the groundwork for a fun-filled childhood, often overseen by the Frazer family's nanny. The Frazers' garden was an adventure wonderland for Ian, his siblings and their friends. A swing and sandpit took centre stage, and Keith and Gerrard both remember the day Sam Frazer arrived home carrying a big, inflatable pool. The Frazers were early adopters of anything new and the first in the neighbourhood also to buy a fridge. The children would line up to receive the ice lollies handed out by Marion. Braid Hills, which was one of the city's summits and offered wonderful views across Edinburgh, could be cold, windy, and sometimes miserable, but the children were oblivious to the temperature, playing in the pool in all weather, whiling away the hours, and eating frozen juice cubes.

Sam worked hard but allowed himself hobbies too, and on non-work days he would feed his passion for cars (the chassis of an Alvis lay in the backyard).

Ian always seemed older than his years. He spoke in phrases that Keith and Gerrard didn't always understand, which on some occasions amused their parents. He was like an adult in some ways; he could be fun, but also serious and determined. Once he started something, whether it was playing the recorder or collecting stamps, he would stick at it in a way many other children could not. Keith discovered this about his friend one day when the two of them had a chat about the big brick wall that stood between their two gardens. The wall had been built in 1952 by Keith's father, and Ian wondered whether it would be possible to make a hole through it using nothing more than metal spoons. Eight hours later, and with a focus beyond their years, they could make out life on the other side of the fence. Eureka! The two eight-year-olds were able to spy on each other through a tiny hole that would remain in the wall for forty years. They had successfully built their own surveillance device. It was an early pointer to a determination that would colour Ian's life and work. In retrospect, it was also a small window into how the need to build would influence him. Whether it was in a sandpit as a toddler, a train set in primary school, a computer software program or kitchen recipe when he was a bit older, he saw success in making a complete whole from many parts, in making a spy hole from a few scratches in a brick wall.

Marion and Sam don't remember Ian's first school day. Like everything else, it was dealt with as matter-of-fact. Ian got up, got dressed and went off without a fuss. Homework happened the same way and Ian quickly excelled, jumping an infant class at George Watson's College. At home, his parents were stern and sometimes even formal. The young clan was required to adhere to strict bedtimes, not fidget at the meal table, speak in a controlled manner, and always display good manners. Their father was a busy man, with big decisions on his plate, and he encouraged the independence Ian showed as an infant. In some ways their father's attitude made the children try harder; they wanted his positive feedback. Sam collected stamps at international conferences to add to Ian's collection and passed on his passion for science as well, luring his eldest to the lab to take blood from him (and diagnosing a condition that had put Ian in bed for a couple of weeks), and leaving science magazines around the family home.

Kirsten, one of the family's nannies, helped grow the fascination all the children showed in science too. As well as taking the youngsters to nearby Braidburn park, so they could clamber around the open-air theatre pretending they were on stage, she also painstakingly made maps of the solar system, and stuck them on their walls. Ian loved it. His interest in science only increased when Sam was appointed professor of chemical pathology at Aberdeen University and the family moved again, firstly to a small rented house nestled between the greengrocer and the local hardware store, and then to a grand old home called Murdan, eight kilometres from the town centre. Sitting well back from Dalmuinzie Road, the huge Victorian home boasted twenty-six rooms and huge gardens. Each of the Frazer children was allowed to choose the colour of the wallpaper for their bedroom. Bought for a song because it was considered at the time to be unfashionably far from town, Murdan would be home to Ian and his siblings through their adolescence.

The broader world the Frazer children were growing into was opening up like a flower too. The Beatles broke into the American music scene with more than seventy million viewers tuning in to a television appearance in 1964, and their hit 'I Want to Hold Your Hand' opened the way for a string of other British artists – from The Rolling Stones to Petula Clark – to dominate the American charts. Cassius Clay changed his name to Muhammad Ali while making boxing popular, the bikini hit the fashion pages and First Lady Jackie Kennedy introduced the world to the pillbox hat. Things weren't as bright in Scotland, which had relied strongly on heavy industry to bolster the economy and was now trying to find something new for its working class. In university circles, academics tried to separate Scotland from Britain in the eyes of the Scottish, but it didn't wash. Unemployment figures rose and infrastructure growth fell. Aberdeen was faring better than other areas, but none of this social upheaval was too obvious in the Frazer household.

It was during their adolescence in Aberdeen that the personalities of the Frazer children started to shine. To both parents, Ian was slightly harder to decipher than Neil, their middle boy, who was softer but the most gregarious – and probably the cheekiest – of their children. Neil gave his parents more trouble than the others too: one night they found the sleepwalker perched at the top of a big open Victorian window. Ewan, their youngest, was obsessed with electronics and managed to make his bedroom door and curtains open by remote control. The young boy's love of technology was fed by his father, whose homemade creations ranged from motorised Daleks, to saws, drills, and skis. In fact, Sam Frazer loved rebuilding cars so much that he bought an old Rolls-Royce just after the Second World War, stripped it down to a pile of scrap metal, and then rebuilt it before travelling around the country to meet other Rolls-Royce enthusiasts.

Much later, Ian would rely on his father's help to build a car from two old vehicles: the first, an Austin A30 bought for thirty quid, was in such poor condition, rusted through, that you could see the ground through the floor. Ian drove it for three years while at university but during that time he and his father put two cars together, managing to weld a new engine into the A30's old engine space. Ian's memory of the project is vivid, and he still bears the scar from dropping the engine on his thumb. That was during the Christmas holidays in his second year of university, but Ian's passion for building would later see him build a computer, write software, and publish a program to make money. Further down the track, with three small children, he would add a room and a deck to their home, and at work he would spend years planning to build the biggest science facility of its kind in the southern hemisphere.

Ian's interest in mechanics was obvious early. As Ewan's life revolved around electronics, Ian would pull things apart and put them back together. All three boys loved their father's train set, which had been housed in the dining room of their Edinburgh house. It would fold down from the wall onto the table. Together they would make tunnels and watch the train whiz through them, over and over again. The boys were only allowed to play with it when Sam was home and they would look forward to seeing their father reach for it.

Ian also shared some of Neil's broader interests. He rode his bicycle for hours at a time, created plastic figurines, and loved music. He was a good child, quiet and serious, who would help his mother with his younger siblings, but as he travelled from infancy through early primary school and into high school, the adjective consistently used to describe him was 'independent'. He relished his own company and from the age of five showed enormous self-confidence. While he didn't boast a lot of friends, he didn't mind, and, while he welcomed praise from his father, he rarely looked to peers to feed his self-approval. It was another character trait, set early.

Ian's sister, Lesley, was a lovely mix of all three of her brothers' personalities. She wore a furrowed brow often, as though she had the weight of the world on her shoulders, but she was feminine too. She fitted in with her brothers: her passion for electronics and science was also obvious from a young age. But her early death, at the age of just ten, tore a hole in the family, stealing the certainty that had marked the children's lives thus far, and creating a void that neither her parents nor her siblings found easy to talk about.

Lesley lost her life in March 1965, on a busy road near the family home. The day had started like any other, with buses ferrying children and parents on the journey in and out of town. Lesley was crossing a two-lane highway, watching the racing traffic, and choosing her moment to get from one side to the other. But it didn't work out. A bus was travelling in one direction and a car in another. Lesley was hit, and died. And so did a part of Sam and Marion. They had been gifted with an easy love, a smooth marriage, and four well-behaved and intelligent children. They lived in a grand old house, had a solid family income, and life had been both good and predictable.

With their daughter's death, all that changed in an instant. Sam and Marion's grief was unimaginable, and they struggled to talk about it, to each other and to their children. For weeks, it seemed to the young boys, the evening meal was eaten in silence as their parents struggled to deal with the loss of their only daughter. Ian, Neil, and Ewan didn't know what to think, and seeing how difficult it was for their parents, they weren't sure where they could turn. Sam and Marion decided the children were too young to attend their sister's funeral, and tears rarely flowed. Eventually Marion told the boys that Lesley would not be returning. It was a short conversation, their mother stating the obvious, but they needed to hear it. Each of the brothers was left to deal with it in his own way – in their bedrooms, in the silence of the Aberdeen nights.

Each day the boys would venture past Lesley's vacant bedroom, a reminder of life gone. Neil remembers his stomach churning the day it was suggested that he move into her room. It was filled with the memory of Lesley and her things were still in place. He hated the idea, but he did it, and it was that move that helped the family to heal. It made it easier for the boys to adjust. Life went on, and, while Lesley's death was always present for her parents, it was rarely talked about. Years later, Neil's wife, Sharon, would only learn about his lost sister after being married for two years. And while Ian's wife, Caroline, was told of the death by others, she only heard it from her husband when he was required, on a visa application, to nominate all siblings, dead or alive.

It was the first time Ian had lost anyone close to him. The predictability of his young life had been stolen in a traffic accident and although he didn't know it then, it would happen to him again, down the track.

Two

It was in the Scottish highlands around Aberdeen that Ian earned his first weekly pay packet, totalling seven quid. On the brink of turning fourteen, he took pride in needing his own national insurance number to join the driven grouse beaters walking the hillsides, waving flags, and sounding horns as shooters, often from England's upper class, tried their luck tagging dinner. The grouse bird is similar to the partridge and served traditionally during the hunting season, which starts in August each year. Grouse beaters herd the birds across heather moors, encouraging them to fly in a direction that allows hunters to target them. Ian loved the job: it was his first real exercise in independence, away from the family home. He welcomed the solitude that came with distance and looked forward to the long hillside walks, a passion that he would feed time and again, later in life. He even loved the risk that came with grouse beating, which meant that if the hunter missed the bird, and got the grouse beater, they were immediately required to hand over a penalty of five quid. Ian was only hit once with a pellet from a 12-bore shotgun, but the shooters never quibbled; some of them were just awful shots, others had indulged in too many drinks. Ian learnt to love cooking during the hunting seasons, camping out and making hot porridge early each morning. But he also learnt quickly to chat up the New Zealand girls who ran the lodge for the shooters, in the hope they would provide him with the leftover dinners.

At school, the young teenager continued to be drawn into the world of science, and astronomy was his subject of choice, perhaps driven by the space race between the Soviet Union and the United States or by his father's subscription to *New Scientist* magazine. The world around him was changing in so many ways, and science was playing a greater role in world affairs.

He was only a youngster, but Ian couldn't ignore talk about the Cuban Missile Crisis, when, for thirteen tense days in October 1962 the Soviet Union and Cuba clashed with the United States. The shipyards of Aberdeen had been bombed during the Second World War, and local talk during the Cuban nuclear crisis centred around fallout and the impact of a bomb potentially hitting Aberdeen. Like many of his peers, he was scared but intrigued, and it further fed his science diet, particularly physics and chemistry. He started learning Russian too, loved English, and pleaded with his parents to study music. They refused that request, preferring that he focus on the more academic subjects; their decision would later influence Ian to encourage his own children to include music in their interests.

Despite his effortless good grades, school was not a natural playground for the adolescent Ian or his brothers. Robert Gordon's College was named after a local merchant who made his money from trading with Baltic ports, and the school carried the Latin motto *omni nunc arte magistra*, meaning 'now is the time for all your masterly skills'. For many of the students, those skills lay on the rugby field and the cricket pitch and Ian, who reached six foot before he became a teenager, wasn't able to match their athleticism. He came across as gangly and a little bit nerdish. He'd fitted in at Braid Hills, with childhood friends Keith and Gerrard, but his new Aberdeen high school, he thought, didn't look as kindly on newcomers.

At home, the boys mostly kept to themselves, each of them independent with their own interests, but sharing a passion for mechanics, electronics, and music. Ian continued to build anything he could, including his own hi-fi system, soldering bits and pieces onto a circuit board. It was his first year in high school. The three boys attempted to build a radio control system but were all disappointed with the range it offered. Ewan, two years later, put his mind to it in the same way his eldest brother chipped away at projects. Later, he would boast to his two brothers about the system he created, and the range he had managed to pull off. That wasn't the last time his parents would see the competitive streak between their eldest and youngest. Sam and Marion valued highly the ability of children to think and work independently, and were proud that their three boys were managing it so effortlessly.

Mealtimes inside Murdan could be quite formal, with the boys telling their parents about their school day before Sam would rush off, again, to work. But on some evenings, and certainly weekends, music would fill the big old rooms, uniting a family passion. The boys' playroom was a billiard room, where a high lamp swung over the table. An old gramophone stood in the corner, with piles of seventy-eight records given to them by their grandparents. Scottish and Irish music, and anything classical, would play out as everyone relaxed.

'Stop Yer Tickling, Jock' by Scotsmen Harry Lauder and Frank Folley was a favourite, and it would be played over and over on the gramophone in the boys' playroom and on a second, superior one enjoyed by their parents. It had speakers in the living room, as well as the dining room, and music filled the halls in between. Despite not studying music, Ian and Ewan took to the piano, creating a competition, ensuring that music remained a passion that the whole family enjoyed. Science remained the chief interest among the brothers, though, cultivated by their parents. Medical journals lay around the house and, like most young boys, the photographs took them in: people with their throats removed, or see-through men and women, highlighting the roles of bones and muscles and ligaments. Presents were tailored to the recipient, and books on science were prized Christmas gifts.

Family holidays were special and involved both camping trips and jaunts to the beach in Italy, where the teenagers tasted real peaches, ice-cream, and spaghetti for the first time. But it wasn't long before Sam and Marion realised that their three fair sons had little interest in the hot Italian beach weather, and the family turned to the snow – sparking Ian's life-long passion for skiing.

The first substantial skiing holiday was to Berwang, a tiny Austrian village close to the German border. Along with studying Russian, Ian had taken up German at school, and to improve his use of it his parents made him arrange the holiday, booking both the accommodation and the lessons. They had skied previously, but only on the basic ski fields close to their home in Aberdeen; a privilege that came with their two shillings and six pence annual subscription to the Alford Ski Club. There, weekend after weekend, Ian would latch himself to a rope attached to a tractor that would pull the skiers up the hill, so they could race down and join the queue for the tractor rope all over again. Ian and his brothers loved the freedom and speed of skiing; their parents were relieved the boys had found a sport they enjoyed and which provided them with good exercise. For three years, they returned to Berwang, taking lessons from Austrian ski instructors, and competing with each other to dominate the easy runs.

It was also on the slopes of Berwang that Ian met Matthias Pirschel, a German teenager just six months older than him. Matthias loved the snow, and Ian loved his company. Apart from the couple of students he learnt Russian with at school, and a few of the science students, Ian didn't have a long list of friends, and he and Matthias became pals, spending the holiday in the snow, and remaining pen pals through their final school years. Matthias's parents worked for the Porsche company in Stuttgart and, after his holiday job as a grouse beater, it was here that Ian took his next holiday job.

To Ian, these three months before he began at The University of Edinburgh represented his first real freedom as a young adult. It involved air travel and visas, paying tax and speaking in German. Everyone and everything seemed so different from Aberdeen, which had yet to open up with the discovery of North Sea oil the following decade. And he marvelled at how different the two countries were.

The automobile industry might have been the jewel in Stuttgart's crown, but the cosmopolitan lifestyles that had seeped in from France and America postwar made Scotland look staid. Ian loved his homeland, but Aberdeen seemed dull beside the bright lights of Germany. In reality, the differences were magnified by the solid and protective home life he had enjoyed. Now he had more questions than answers. He was upset, as an atheist, to be forced to pay a church tax in Germany. He was also upset when his first real girlfriend dumped him. But with each closing door, another opened, and he immersed himself in a world outside Aberdeen.

By the end of his stay, he was fluent in German and even dreamt in German. His language skills, and obvious intelligence, also provided his first promotion: he was put in charge of the factory's metallurgy laboratory when the boss went on holiday. Ian was just seventeen, and he took it seriously, calmly dealing with irate German suppliers who had sent flawed components to the factory and had them returned. Ian applied a simple rule, in the same way he often saw things as black and white: if the components did not meet the specifications, he would reject them, and he continued to do that, shocking many when they asked to speak to his boss.

These formative experiences in Germany ensured that he returned during future university summer holidays, working in various jobs, from a government institute set up to house problem drinkers away from hotels, to working in a pub where he only received payment from the angry hotelier if Ian could stop his wife from making herself sick on cheap wine, to working as a chef in a small German town. And through it, Matthias and Ian remained friends, enjoying each other's company, and occasionally holidaying together.

Indeed, it was during one of these camping trips – when Matthias was off with his girlfriend, Doris – that Ian decided how he wanted to spend his life. In a life of milestones, this was an important one: a conversation that would help Ian focus on where he was going, and turn him in another direction.

His natural intelligence had allowed him to amble down the road of physics, which he loved. Now, away from his home and with Matthias focused on his girlfriend, Ian was left to chat to her father, a professor. He listened as Ian tried to articulate his future, and his love of physics. But as Ian said it, the words didn't ring true to him. He had avoided medicine, his father's field. Independence had dictated that he, like most teenagers, wanted to do something other than what his parents had chosen. But now, sitting alongside a man he hardly knew, he realised physics wasn't right. He made the decision, on the spot, to focus on medicine instead.

It was a seminal moment for Ian, putting him on the path to study immunology, a science that would later lead to a cure for the virus that causes cervical cancer. Ironically, it was Ian's father, whose footsteps he had tried not to trace, who had to then help ensure that his eldest son gained a spot in the faculty of medicine. Ian wasn't sure whether a few strings were pulled or not, but he was interviewed and formally accepted to study medicine at The University of Edinburgh. Cambridge had been his first choice, but he'd failed the entrance exam, courtesy of a disjoined curricula across regions, meaning the young scholar from Robert Gordon's College in Aberdeen could top the country in physics but be stopped from walking through the door of his chosen university.

Three

The dead body of a woman, aged about sixty, lay out on the table in front of them. David Henry Gillespie, Robin Cregeen and Ian Frazer peered over her left side. Another three anatomy students stood on the other side of the table. The hall was strewn with forty similar bodies, each lying on its own table and placed two metres apart. The second-year University of Edinburgh medical students had been divided into teams of three, and each given one side of a body. Over the next fifteen months it was their task to learn as much as possible about the 'patient'. They were required to dissect it, starting with the arms, then the chest, the abdomen, and the legs. Robin hated the idea so much that he skipped the class a few times; the idea of carving up a body did not sit easily with him. David didn't want to be there either, and both he and Robin were incredulous at the way their friend went about the class. Ian Frazer was focused and serious and meticulous, following instructions and building on the knowledge that came with them. He wanted to understand each new complication and work out the answer. Robin and David wanted to bolt from the room, and they thanked their lucky stars that Ian was on their team.

Robin had met the tall Scotsman during freshers' week the previous year. They had completed their first introductory medical school meeting and were waiting in a queue. Robin was reading a magazine called *Synapse* and made reference to it. Ian, in his strong Scottish brogue, hit back at his pronunciation of the title, correcting him. But the way he did it didn't offend Robin in the slightest. It was without malice, and they struck up an easy conversation. David, an archetypal kilt-wearing redhead, was also in their class and his chance meeting with Ian happened a few months later over coffee and a crossword in the university canteen. He marvelled at Ian's abilities too: he'd solved the crossword in a matter of minutes, spoke fluent German, and talked about tinkering with cars. It all seemed to come as easily as it looked for Ian.

Despite a bout of glandular fever in his first year, Ian's physics, chemistry, and biology subjects mirrored much of the curriculum he had undertaken in his final year at school. Living in the student hall at Edinburgh University, he felt at home. He didn't need to walk to anyone else's tune. He happily trotted off to lectures in sandals that many thought were a bit unfashionable. He studied what he had to, generous with his knowledge and aware that he seemed to do less work than many of his colleagues. And with a newfound independence, he packed his free time with his passions of music and organising skiing trips.

Eventually Ian moved out of university accommodation and into a flat with David in Livingston, twenty-five kilometres west of Edinburgh University. Music filled the cheap little unit. Ian still had his A30, and later a mini-van, and the pair would travel to Edinburgh each day for lectures. Life revolved around home brew and fondue and they took turns cooking, laughing at the curries with a touch too much chilli, and hosting parties well into the night. David says now that he probably should have spent more time studying while living with Ian; it took him too long to learn that Ian could get remarkable grades by doing half the amount of work that others required. But he thought he might have had the edge when it came to music.

It was their interest in music that was behind their mobile disco business. Ian built an amplifier and loudspeaker cabinets and the pair used their domestic record players, bought cheap flashing lights, and set out to earn a bit of cash working in private homes and small halls providing the music for disco nights. The Rolling Stones featured strongly in their set list. Neither of them enjoyed the DJ chat between songs, so record after record was played without a break.

Later they moved together to another flat, where they were always quick to get home from class for a filtered coffee and to watch television late into the night or make the most of cheap concert tickets for the Scottish National Orchestra playing in the Usher Hall, just up the road. And every weekend possible, Ian would escape to the snow, spending hours skiing and, at one stage, even wondering whether he could make a quid as an instructor.

Which is precisely what he did over the Easter break in 1975; he organised a university skiing trip to Mürren, a Walser mountain village in Switzerland. A big group of students stayed in the Grand Chalet, a pretty timber lodge with high icing-sugar snow-capped eaves. Everyone slept in dormitory accommodation, with the girls supposed to sleep on one floor and boys on the other, although that didn't always happen.

Communal washrooms were located on each floor, and the big dining room and kitchen were located downstairs.

The chalet sauna was popular after a day on the slopes, and Carol Collee, a close friend remembers one particular day when Ian was in there naked. Carol and another student sat alongside him. Saunas were just starting to appear in Edinburgh, and the fashion set talked about their European colleagues jumping from sauna into snow to make snow angels. Ian never looked cutting edge, but he was up with the latest trends. Carol had met the tall Scotsman with the distinctive walk and talk the previous year when he dropped into her medical class. She thought he was brilliant academically but seemed modest too – not that you'd know now, sitting naked in the sauna a world away from Edinburgh University. But Carol, still a close friend, knew early on that Ian never sought validation from anyone. 'It's not important to him if people think he is wearing the right attire,' she says, 'or the right shoes, or says the right thing. He'll go with protocol, but he doesn't look for approval.'

Carol had come as one of four chalet girls, who were allowed to ski for free in return for feeding the big hungry group. She loved it. She and the forty other Edinburgh University Ski Club members just had to turn up to the bus with a sleeping bag, and Ian Frazer had done the rest. He had booked the overnight bus to London, the cross-channel ferry to Calais, the train to Interlaken, and the funicular railway that snaked up to the chalet door, organising passports, border control, lift passes, and accommodation. He'd managed to plan the logistics for the whole trip between classes.

Carol says he also dealt with two worrying incidents on the trip: when one passenger became lost, and when another fell very sick. Ian acted quickly on both occasions, taking over police discussions in the first instance, and diagnosing the student with spontaneous pneumothorax and arranging a transfer to the local hospital in the second case. Pneumothorax is a condition that needs medical attention very quickly. It can hit fit young males when they go up to high altitudes, causing one of the air sacs in the lung to burst and subsequently collapse.

Most afternoons, after taking calculated risks on snow runs for hours each day, Ian would relax in the sauna. And then, with all the other students, he would settle back in the chalet to make flagons of mulled wine to go with the spaghetti bolognaise, chicken casserole, or shepherd's pie that would inevitably be prepared by Carol and her friends. Ian had turned twenty-two, but appeared years older than many of his peers. He laughed and drank, just as they did, but he always managed to escape being the centre of attention. When the food fights got out of hand, Ian could be found watching from the sideline. The fondue parties ended with big hangovers and it was Ian who would knock on the door early the next day with his secret hangover cure. (Carol believed it included alcohol and soluble paracetamol; Ian, with a cheeky grin, always maintained it was simply orange juice and soda water.)

Ian was again on the sidelines on the day a group of lads took their kilts to the top of a snow run, bared their butts, and then removed their kilts. In those days streaking was not very common and considered a bit naughty. Everyone laughed, and Ian joined in, fully dressed. A similar thing happened one night at the Stager Stubli restaurant, or the Stagger Stumble as the students called it, when an alcohol-fuelled snow fight broke out. Everyone joined in, and everyone was evicted. But later, many of them realised that Ian had left just before the trouble started, tucking himself into bed as others were ordered out of the restaurant. He also escaped the outbreak of cold sores and herpes that hit some of the snow's revellers; his only interest in that was viral epidemiology.

It was later in the same year – 1975 – with a Bachelor of Science in pathology already in his top drawer, that Ian made a decision that would shift his career path again. Still just twenty-two years old, he joined the Australian working visa scheme, travelling to Australia as an intern at the Walter and Eliza Hall Institute of Medical Research in Melbourne. The visa scheme was a means of attracting mining students to the faraway land, but a token collection of other students were allowed too. Ian had just done an immunology project as an honours student in pathology. Every way he turned, the Walter and Eliza Hall Institute of Medical Research sprang up. Ian liked its emphasis on immunology; he also liked that it was on the other side of the world.

After accepting a wage of twenty dollars a week (a stipend had to be paid to students joining the scheme) and under the supervision of John Mathews at the institute, Ian began his eight-week stint in the land he would later call home. Housed in the students' quarters at the Royal Melbourne Hospital, Ian worked hard and enjoyed the hospitality of Mathews and his family on weekend trips to the Dandenong Ranges. Mathews thought the young student stood out from the crowd of students, with his inquiring mind and organisational skills. Most of Ian's projects involved vasectomies and high blood pressure, and he went about his work methodically, asking all the right questions and impressing Mathews time and again. They developed an easy friendship, playing chess and talking about science. In a stroke of luck, Mathews introduced the Scottish student to Ian Mackay, who headed the clinical research unit at the Royal Melbourne Hospital and the corresponding department at the institute.

Mackay was a demanding boss, and prickly to some too. He wanted to get the best out of his researchers, and challenged them often. He also ran a traditional hospital ward round, which started each day on the dot of 9 a.m. Punctuality was important, and, as the students, residents, registrar, and visiting consultants followed him, Mackay would throw them questions to test their understanding. First, he would see if the students could answer the question; if not, he would ask the medical residents, then the registrar and, finally, the visiting consultants. Often, only Ian Mackay would know the correct answer.

Ian Frazer was both punctual and interested and would often turn up at the institute's lunchtime seminars to learn something new. On his last Friday, Ian Mackay asked him to present on the differences between being a medical student in Australia and Scotland. Ian delivered his talk with gusto, and then set off to see other parts of the big new country he knew he would visit again one day.

But there was a reason Ian was also keen to go home quickly, and he was counting down the days until he arrived back in Scotland. Her name was Caroline Nicoll, and he had met her two years earlier, in her first year studying at Edinburgh University. She was outgoing and funny and opinionated and sporty. And no one else quite had his measure. He couldn't get her out of his head.

Four

Caroline Jane Robertson Nicoll noticed his blue eyes first. She'd never seen eyes quite that colour before. It was February 1973, and the busload of skiers was winding its way up to Aviemore, a three-hour trip from Edinburgh University. Caroline was sitting down the back next to Lesley Buchanan, who was also in her first year of a Bachelor of Education. Caroline was majoring in maths and biology; Lesley's focus lay in physics and maths. They both loved sport and would frequently team up to play squash. But on this day, they had joined the university ski club for its first weekend away. The tall third-year student, who had organised the trip, was hunched over talking to someone a few rows in front, but it was hard to miss those eyes, as well as the blue beanie he was wearing.

Caroline Nicoll watched as Ian Frazer moved to the next row of skiers, talking to new recruits about what to expect, and answering questions posed by others. He looked like a pretty cool character, she thought. Eventually he got to the back row, where she sat with Lesley, and they started talking. She found herself drawn to him instantly; he didn't mind the look of her friend Lesley.

The weekend was a wonderful escape from Edinburgh, and Caroline, a talented sportswoman who had only been skiing twice before, and Lesley mixed and mingled, meeting other university students across courses and years. The accommodation was cheap and cold, but the students stayed up late, dining and dancing. Ian stuck in Caroline's mind, and with Lesley showing no interest in him, Ian soon found himself spending big chunks of the weekend talking to the young woman who was born in Perth, between Edinburgh and Dundee in Scotland, in October 1954. She liked a challenge, he could tell that, and the next day, as weary skiers boarded the bus, he unknowingly delivered her one.

There were two ways of descending the mountain: one was by bus, the way they had arrived; the other was to ski down and meet the bus at the bottom. It wasn't an easy run, night was closing in, and no ski patrols were monitoring the slopes. One by one, Ian selected who could keep their skis on, and travel down by themselves, and who would be directed to travel by bus because he was not confident they were experienced enough for the alternative. He neither entertained arguments, nor cared about who he offended in making the decision. He was in charge, and everyone just seemed to accept that.

Ian pointed to Lesley, Caroline's friend, and indicated that she was able to join the experienced skiers and meet the bus at the bottom of the mountain. He then asked Caroline to board the bus. Caroline shot back quickly, questioning him. He told her straight – she was not yet good enough to take on this run. She boarded the bus and took her seat in silence. No one had ever told her that she wasn't quite good enough for something, and she didn't like it. The next time she joined a club trip there would be no doubting her skiing ability: she would ski with the others down the mountainside. Caroline was miffed, and Ian saw it. He started to wonder a bit more about her.

A few days later, he tracked her down and asked her to one of his mobile disco parties. He also asked her to bring Lesley, a request that Caroline forgot to pass on to her friend. Caroline thought that she would spend the night dancing and getting to know the third-year medical student who seemed to dabble in everything. But from the start, nothing went to plan. David Gillespie was responsible for the party's music, and when someone spilled beer over the amplifier quick action was needed. Ian jumped in his car, Caroline in the passenger side, to source a new loudspeaker or parts. Their hunt lasted a few hours before they gave it up, and she never made it to the party, or to dance.

Caroline went home happy that night knowing that she had learnt more about Ian, but was still disappointed it hadn't been the night she had thought it would be. Ian felt bad too; he was interested in the gregarious and pretty woman who had taken a liking to him, and he promised to make it up to her with a picnic in the woods the following day. On impulse, she agreed, and the next day Ian and Caroline shared a black forest gateau and a bottle of wine in the woods at Penicuik, about twelve kilometres outside of Edinburgh. They talked about themselves and university and discovered they both liked music and walking. From that day it was a relaxed pairing, filled with common interests. Skiing became one, but so too did classical music, and, with Ian a subscriber of the Scottish National Orchestra, it wasn't long before Caroline joined Ian and his friend David Gillespie as semi-regulars in the cheap seats.

Caroline's influence over Ian was marked and immediate. She was natural and lively and chatty and sporty, able to mix easily with everyone, and everyone seemed to love her. Ian felt proud of that, and quickly became protective. He loved that he could talk to her in a way that perhaps he hadn't been able to talk with anyone else previously. Ian's vast general knowledge and enviable ability to succeed at whatever he tried meant that people rarely disagreed with him. Caroline didn't have any of that reverence. She was taken by his intelligence and his love of music, but she also thought he was fun and interesting: she liked the whole package. The blue eyes his mother had first noticed, and that Caroline had first seen on their skiing trip, continued to captivate her. They saw each other often, and exclusively.

But after several months, Caroline began to have a rethink. She was a first-year student, spending all her free time with her new boyfriend. They were invited places together, not separately. She really liked him, but wondered whether it was all happening too quickly. She worried that she was too young and that their relationship had gone from casual to serious overnight. She didn't quite know what to do, but ended up telling Ian that she wanted a break.

He didn't show it, but he was devastated. He was besotted with her, and took her decision to break up with him hard. He dragged himself around, going to lectures, joining his friends over coffee, getting on with life but without the spark that marked his usual wit. David, his best friend and flatmate, saw it, and so did his mother. Caroline wasn't enjoying the break much either.

Three weeks later Ian decided to visit Caroline, taking back a book she had left at his home. He knocked on her door, and she let him in. It reignited both their romance and Ian's spark, and restarted a relationship that would become his greatest partnership and achievement.

It was following a two-month holiday driving across Europe that cemented their future. Without a radio in their little mini-van, they talked and talked. Science was rarely, if ever, mentioned, and they spent their days walking and wandering around ancient sites. Ian had never met anyone whose company he enjoyed more; Caroline learnt more about Ian too, especially his ability to remain calm in any situation. Caroline tells the story of when they nearly ran out of petrol on top of a pass heading towards Italy. Ian decided to turn off the mini-van's engine to conserve fuel. As they hurtled around hairpin bends, Caroline grew terrified. She looked across at Ian, who remained unruffled – a personality trait she has long admired.

By the time Ian left for his student trip to the Walter and Eliza Hall Institute in Melbourne in 1975, they both knew they would marry. But Ian left nothing to chance. He suggested to Caroline that she take a job as an auxiliary nurse at a hospital, so she would know what it was like to be married to a doctor. She loved it, and, given an earlier experience she'd had studying biology, this was welcome.

Back in second year, Caroline was required to complete a project which involved measuring and weighing a mouse daily. But each time she entered the lab, she would find another baby mouse dead, a stray claw or tail the only evidence it had been there the previous day. Caroline started to dread going in, and confided in Ian. His answer, as always, was swift and definite: Caroline's handling of the mouse meant its mother rejected it, and then ate it. He said he would deal with the dead mice, and she loved him for it. But she wasn't blinded by her love for Ian. Just as Robin Cregeen, who had mispronounced the name of a science magazine, felt Ian Frazer's abrupt but honest disregard for tact, Caroline sometimes felt it too. On one occasion she had her hair cut for the medical faculty ball she was attending as Ian's partner. Dressed to the nines and feeling proud of herself, Caroline knocked on his door. 'You look like a boy,' he said, after opening it. Caroline refused to speak to him all night. From then on, Ian learnt to be more careful in phrasing his comments.

Throughout their courtship, and until they married a month after her graduation in July 1976, Caroline lived with seven other girls, all sharing one bathroom. It was a big happy house that she had moved into after living with her aunt during her first year at university. Now with her Bachelor of Education completed, the couple planned to marry. Caroline would take up an offer to teach high-school maths across town from the university, while Ian would continue his study ahead of his graduation the following year, in June 1977.

The Frazers loved Caroline from the moment their son brought her back to the family's Aberdeen home one weekend, early in their courtship. Marion went to bed thinking that her son had found the perfect partner: Caroline was attractive and athletic and kind, and they obviously loved each other's company. Caroline would be good for their eldest son, she 'thought. Caroline liked them too, but she found herself fearing Sam Frazer on some occasions. He was quiet and stern, and certainly very bright. Neither of her parents had been to university.

The Nicolls liked Ian too, but had reservations about their daughter walking up the aisle at the age of twenty-one. As Caroline's family sat in the kitchen of their home in Perth, Ian told her parents he wanted to marry her. Caroline, with her ear to the wall, listened from next door. Hearing Ian ask for his daughter's hand in marriage, Caroline's father, John, saw it as inevitable, and was quite phlegmatic about it. Ian was obviously very clever, perhaps even a bit academic, but they were also unsure of his prospects. Ian had an answer: once he graduated he would be busy with work, and he and Caroline wanted to organise themselves and a household together before life became too busy. This was for both of them. Ian walked out with a firm seal of approval. Caroline, still with her ear to the wall next door, was delighted.

Scotland's drought ended, and the heavens opened, at 3 p.m. one Saturday in July 1976. Carrying yellow and white roses, Caroline wore a long white dress she had found while shopping with her mother. Her bridesmaids, including Lesley Buchanan, wore early daffodil yellow Laura Ashley dresses. Ian and his groomsmen – his brothers and David Gillespie – wore hired family kilts before the Presbyterian minister. It was a practical, pretty, and traditional wedding, which respected Caroline's parents' wishes. The vows were taken in Kinnoull Parish Church before the reception at the Hunting Tower House Hotel, on the outskirts of Perth. Ian gave a short speech, thanking the bridesmaids. Caroline's father loathed speaking publicly and handed the responsibility over to her uncle, who coped, despite not knowing the young bride particularly well. Her second cousin helped out by making the three-tiered wedding cake. In fact, the day only went off script when the Jack Russell belonging to Marion's sister escaped from the car and chased a paddling of ducks up a tree.

The honeymoon spent camping around the north of Scotland was short and Ian and Caroline quickly settled into domestic life. Each morning Caroline would rise early to travel across town by bus to teach at Firrhill Comprehensive School in Edinburgh's south-west. Ian focused on the last year of his medical degree, toiling away at university between frequent skiing trips. Together they made a home in a cheap and dingy little apartment, in a big, grey, stone building right beside a graveyard. In fact, the top of their bed butted up against the solid graveyard wall. It was a very humble start, but they both felt as if they owned the world.

Five

Caroline was home on a Monday night in January 1978 when her husband walked through the door looking like he'd been put through a wringer. Adept at not showing emotion, he couldn't escape her watchful eye and she knew something was dreadfully wrong. And it was. 'They keep dying,' he told his young wife. 'Everybody is dying.'

In four days, Ian Frazer had lost thirteen patients in his care. He'd only graduated as a doctor from The University of Edinburgh a year earlier. His first work placement was as a house officer at Roodlands Hospital in Haddington, where he did a bit of everything, including surgery, but now he was house officer at Eastern General, a much bigger hospital. Here he held more responsibility, and a position equivalent to that of medical resident. He was highly regarded and worked hard, sometimes doing his ward rounds without a nurse. This was an unusual practice for someone of Ian's limited experience, but he was confident and quickly won over patients' respect and affection. He also shone at interdepartmental meetings, prompting one of his student colleagues to dub him the 'medical ballet dancer'. The nickname stuck as he presented clinical cases with a polished elegance that many of his peers couldn't match. His superiors watched the jealous reaction of one student colleague to Ian's rising star. But Ian was oblivious to the bait being served up, or he ignored it. Either way, his bosses noted that Ian never gave ground and seemed to be the conciliatory force among the group of talented young doctors.

But this Monday afternoon, none of that seemed to be true. He was exhausted, and Caroline could see it. It was the middle of winter and his shift had started on Thursday and ended on Monday. Patients had died at regular intervals over those few days, despite Ian's best attempts. Of course, death in this ward was not uncommon because many of the patients arrived very ill with chronic bronchitis. But Ian thought he must have done something dreadfully wrong. He had always been able to come up with an answer. Things had always seemed to work out. But now, in front of him, patients were dying one after another. They had come into a big hospital expecting to get better. Their brothers and sisters and children wore expectation on their faces, and he felt responsible for disappointing them. He had to sit down and explain to these families that their loved one was dead. It was depressing, particularly the case of one young man. He had a nasty vasculitis, an inflammation of the blood vessels, which had not been picked up earlier, and by the time he reached a bed at the Eastern General, it was too late. Ian knew that this could happen, that hospitals cared for dangerously ill patients, but the spate of deaths in such a short time affected him.

He and his doctor colleagues usually dealt with patient deaths through black humour. If a deceased patient needed cremating, the doctor on duty had to fill out a form, certifying the patient was dead and what the cause of death had been. This prompted a fee, or 'cremmy money' as the doctors would call it, and it would arrive in brown paper bags from the man who ran the funeral parlour. This weekend, Ian's fellow residents felt that he had cheated them out of their share because many of the dead had been their patients during the week. Ian had walked away with a healthy bonus and, while it was easy to laugh at the absurdity of the situation, Caroline could see it was playing on her husband's mind. He didn't think it was funny.

From the day Ian was interviewed for the job at Eastern General Hospital, his superiors believed they had snagged a clever young doctor. The job application system was fairly primitive, but those sitting around the table had been impressed by Ian the moment he opened his mouth. He was an innovative thinker and didn't come across as arrogant, but he certainly had confidence in his abilities and capacity to do the job. Just as he had shown business acumen as a student by organising a fully sponsored year book, it stood out that Ian Hector Frazer wasn't like every other applicant applying for a position at Eastern General. His academic achievements, in black and white, stood out, but his performance during the interview was unmatched. He was bright and articulate, with an intelligence that Dr John Munro thought was well beyond his years.

Ian Frazer intrigued Munro, a senior consultant who became one of the young doctor's bosses at Eastern General. He seemed confident in everything he did. He looked the part, despite wearing flip-flop sandals around the ward. In fact, Munro used to wonder whether Ian's feet were so big that sandals were more comfortable, or whether he was unable to afford decent shoes. But he got away with it, because he was popular with staff and patients alike. Tall and gangly, Ian didn't need reassurance on how to dress, or in diagnosing patients. And when he made a mistake, he was quick to put his hand up and learn. Munro, who is still in regular contact with Ian, tagged him as someone who would make a real difference as a medical practitioner.

And that was Ian's intention – to work as a clinical doctor, not a researcher, helping patients by their bedside. He had trained as a doctor, graduated as a doctor and, right up until he was trained as a renal physician, believed he was on the road to becoming a transplant immunologist. But the pull to do research was strong too, and was given a mighty nudge after two stints in the medical renal unit at the Royal Infirmary in Edinburgh.

Ian Frazer joined the renal unit as a senior house officer in 1978 after his time at the Eastern General Hospital, and again in 1980 as a registrar. During both stints, the black cloud that hung over the unit turned his interests elsewhere. The resident psychiatrist was the first person Ian was introduced to; he thought the specialist was there to work with patients, guiding them through the psychological trauma that came with their illness, but soon found out that the bigger chunk of his job related to staff trauma.

Many of the patients were young and chronically ill and in danger of taking their last breath each time they were put on dialysis. This had a dreadful impact on many of the young medicos. Some patients waited and waited for kidney transplants that never arrived because of the shortage of donors. Nothing existed to control the minor metabolites that caused problems for dialysis back then, and one of Ian's patients mirrored a walking exoskeleton: his whole skin was calcified because the doctors had been unable to get his calcium balance right. An outbreak of hepatitis B also caused the death of several patients. Ian and his colleagues did what they could to stay in good spirits and spread a bit of cheer.

One year Ian even dressed up as Santa to deliver presents to the patients and staff, and staff would write and perform a play for patients. But he struggled to like the job, and the pull of research and the questions that immunology posed but couldn't answer continued to grow. He and Caroline talked about his next move, and both were drawn to a PhD in immunology at Cambridge University under Alan Munro, brother of John Munro, Ian's boss at Eastern General Hospital.

When Ian had broached the subject of marriage with Caroline's parents, he'd argued the importance of marrying before he graduated, so they could set up home and be organised. That had proved a good selling point to her parents, and had worked a treat for the newlyweds too. Caroline continued to travel across Edinburgh each day to teach senior maths, and the couple worked hard and saved what they could. Eventually, with their own savings and some help provided by Ian's parents, they bought their own Edinburgh apartment. To buy it they borrowed seventeen thousand pounds.

At home, Ian showed off in the kitchen, quickly becoming skilled at those dishes that drew his attention. Fondues – meat, chocolate and chicken – were all in, and the couple would host dinner parties with friends well into the night, laughter filling their apartment. They lived simply because their incomes didn't really allow for anything else, and most of their savings were directed at skiing trips. Ian bought one suit from Marks and Spencer for his first job interview (and would keep wearing it until he was named Australian of the Year thirty years later), and the old A30 he had built with his father was eventually replaced by the mini-van after Caroline refused to travel in it, fearing they would fall through to the ground they could see through the floor. Money continued to be in short supply for years, but as long as they had enough after paying the grocery bill to escape to the snow for the weekend, they were happy.

In January 1981, they spent a week on the slopes of Val d'Isère in France. With the snow good, and both intent on honing their skiing skills on some of the bigger slopes, they forgot about Edinburgh and what Ian might do next.

The PhD under Alan Munro appealed to Ian for two reasons: John Munro, Alan's brother, had been a mentor and Ian knew that under Munro's supervision he would be challenged and happy. And more and more his interest in immunology was growing. It was an area that needed attention; some claimed all that was known about it could be scribbled on the back of a stamp. It was also unfashionable, a bit unsexy, not that that worried Ian Frazer; in fact the general lack of knowledge in the area actually appealed to him.

With a bag full of dirty clothes and hardly a cent left in the bank, the couple arrived home from France to make their next big decision. Then, in timing that is hard to figure, a telegram arrived addressed to Ian. They held their breaths while they opened it, having never received one before: usually, a telegram signalled terrible news, like a death in the family.

'Where are you?' they read. 'Isn't it time you came back?'

It was signed by Ian Mackay, head of clinical research at the Royal Melbourne Hospital and the Walter and Eliza Hall Institute, who Ian had met when he was first in Australia as a student in 1975. Ian was both relieved the telegram didn't involve a family death, and baffled by its contents. He had been one student five years before at the institute. And while he had been introduced to Ian Mackay and, at his instigation, given a presentation, he didn't think any of it had been a prerequisite for a job. He didn't think he'd left that much of an impression. But the telegram was clear: he was being offered a job on the other side of the world, in Melbourne, Australia.

It was a natural decision. During his study of immunology, research papers kept popping up from the Walter and Eliza Hall Institute. It had an excellent worldwide reputation, and Ian had also seen the work being conducted there firsthand during his eight-week stint at the end of his fourth year. It also provided a timely escape from the Scottish economy, which was struggling under the weight of high unemployment and Margaret Thatcher's early rule: some companies swam, but many sank. With their minds made up virtually in an instant, Alan Munro lost out, and the pair started the long, slow process of obtaining visas for Australia.

The following month, in March 1981, Caroline discovered she was pregnant with their first child. It was a surprise to the couple. They both wanted children, but this had happened faster than they had planned. Caroline learnt of her pregnancy from the doctor who conducted her visa application medical exam. It certainly threw another variable into the mix: they were about to move to another country, where they had no family support. A child, while cherished, would just make it a little busier.

Shortly before they left Scotland, the couple dined with Robin Cregeen, Ian's friend from university, and his wife, Angela, telling them excitedly about their plans. Ian grinned broadly as they parted, and said that he and Caroline would see them in a couple of years. At that stage they planned to return to the United Kingdom to raise their family. They were united in that decision.

A few weeks later – and five years after they were married – Ian and Caroline boarded a plane to begin the journey to their new and temporary Australian home, stopping off in America on the way over. With Caroline suffering dreadful morning sickness, they landed in Melbourne ready for Ian to start work on the first day of May 1981. He was going to be a senior research officer in Ian Mackay's Australian laboratory.

Six

For many, the Melbourne Cup serves as an excellent way of carbon dating our memories, in the same way a big news story is a marker in our lives. We might remember what we wore and where we were when we cheered Makybe Diva across the line three times. Our children have all learnt about Phar Lap and each year the Cup enriches the national folklore. So it was that more than two decades after Tommy Smith's first victory in the Melbourne Cup, Just a Dash made it to the line first. Smith had reportedly had more hope in another one of his horses, but, on this Tuesday afternoon in November 1981, it was this thoroughbred that stormed home. Ian Mackay let out a cheer, joining the chorus of celebration at Flemington, where fashion in the field showed off every style under the sun. Caroline sat in a chair, fanning away the hot wind on her first visit to the infamous horserace. She and Ian had heard about it, but this was their first experience up close. It was a stinking hot day, a few weeks short of 18 November, the day Caroline and Ian Frazer's first child would be born.

It was almost six months to the day since the couple had arrived in Melbourne, and after being put up in temporary accommodation for a few weeks, they now had their own place in Carlton North. The little ground-floor apartment was humble by anyone's standards; the dining and coffee tables and fridge were all rented because they didn't have the cash to buy anything new. Their bed was bought on hire-purchase so eventually they would at least own that. Without a car, they walked everywhere. But the prints on the walls hid their lack of money, courtesy of a local library program that allowed Melbourne residents to borrow copies of the works of famous Australian artists. Ian and Caroline loved it, each month exchanging paintings by Frederick McCubbin or Russell Drysdale.

By Scotland's standards, Melbourne's winter weather was glorious, and each morning when Ian ventured off to work Caroline would wander the wide streets, marvelling at the trams, the choice of local restaurants, and the culture that encouraged people out of their homes. Edinburgh and Melbourne seemed like chalk and cheese, and the local milk bars fascinated her as much as the local lingo, with words like 'arvo', 'veges', and 'smoko' confusing and amusing her. At local parks she would watch young mothers' groups, wondering whether she'd be welcome in a few months' time, and how to meet people in a new country, without a job. It was exciting, but bouts of loneliness and homesickness were common too.

Ian and Caroline believed they were in Australia for a couple of years, not a lifetime, and expected to settle back home eventually. That had made the move easier. The hardest part in leaving, for both of them, had been Caroline's goodbye to her family. While the couple had found out that she was pregnant at the compulsory medical check-up for her Australian visa they had decided not to share the baby news with their families until the pregnancy had progressed. Although Caroline knew that was a sensible thing to do, it left her feeling guilty. She was going to the other side of the world to have each family's first grandchild. At least, she thought, it would provide a good reason for their parents to visit during their Australian sojourn.

Ian had a job, but he certainly wasn't high in the pecking order. In fact, as Ian Mackay's second assistant physician, he was just under the first assistant, Mathew Vadas, and close to the bottom of the pile. It wasn't long before Mathew and Ian were good friends and Mathew and his girlfriend, Jennifer, were introducing their Scottish friends to the ski slopes at Perisher and Thredbo. Caroline felt at home, and despite being seven months' pregnant and unable to do up her ski jacket, she flew down her first Australian ski runs impressed at the winter snowfalls.

Mathew was ten years older than Ian but they liked each other instantly and held a similar view of their boss. Ian Mackay was an interesting character. Early in his career he contracted tuberculosis, which was then treated in a sanatorium. The diagnosis curtailed his medical career for many years and, when fortune swung his way and he managed to get back into the system, the same diagnosis ruled out his dreams of being a chest physician. But another door soon opened, and his work turned to the study of liver disease and eventually to the Walter and Eliza Hall Institute.

Ian Mackay had had his eye on Frazer since the young Scotsman had worked in Melbourne in 1975. Mackay liked him. Frazer was talented, keen on research, diligent, courteous, and never ever late, and that was important to a physician who valued punctuality as Ian Mackay did. Mathew and Ian liked their boss but often felt the full force of his personality. He could be both fatherly and acerbic in a short space of time, and the two young physicians were never sure whether he truly trusted them. Certainly Ian Mackay was protective of his patients and would frequently double-check any diagnosis offered up by Ian or Mathew.

Ian's brief was to work on chronic liver disease, with Mackay strongly interested in autoimmunity and those liver diseases which were driven by the immune system's attacking the liver. The slog was hard and slow, and Ian's attention was diverted from autoimmune liver disease to the chronic active hepatitis caused by hepatitis B virus infection. As he worked away each day, he kept asking himself a question that he could not answer: why were some people who got hepatitis B virus infection able to get rid of it, while others could not?

Outside work, Australia seemed to offer so much more than the smoky, cold confines of Edinburgh. With their new baby girl, Jennifer, they celebrated their first antipodean Christmas in South Australia, where Caroline spent her time pleading with Ian not to go swimming. He ignored those pleas and embraced the sand, sun and surf that he had only heard about in Edinburgh. Caroline had read up on Australia before the move, and sharks had been mentioned frequently. She worried that a great white might be lurking below the pristine waters off the South Australian coast.

Caroline had only nursed a couple of babies before Jennifer turned their world upside down in the most delightful ways. Ian became more talkative at work once Jennifer came along, and over coffee or at home with a bowl of chilli con carne and syllabub, he would entertain his colleagues with stories about each new milestone. He was every bit the proud dad and sometimes he would even disappear home late in the afternoon, his colleagues knowing that when Caroline and Jennifer fell asleep that evening, he would sneak back to work and return to his desk.

Still planning to return to Scotland in two years, Ian and Caroline grabbed the opportunity to see as much of Australia as they could and travelled to the Great Barrier Reef, Uluru, along the Great Ocean Road, and took photographs in the Blue Mountains. The wide open spaces and the differences that lay within the one country captivated them. They had read about it, and now they were seeing it firsthand. Scotland seemed so small in comparison.

Back in Melbourne, they marvelled at apricots growing on trees and the first jacaranda blooms. Skiing remained their winter fun, and, after buying a two-fifths share in a windsurfer, Friday evenings in summer were often spent on Port Phillip Bay catching the perfect wind. Sometimes it was quite dark when they would pack up after windsurfing, often Ian would have to rescue Caroline, who could venture out too far and find herself unable to turn the windsurfer back to shore.

They were enjoying life in Melbourne more and more and starting to cement some close friendships. Paul Andrews had come to Australia with his wife, Trish, shortly after Ian and Caroline had arrived. Paul worked as a biochemist at the institute, looking at an immune organ called the thymus. Located in the chest, the thymus is a seed organ that helps create the immune system. Paul and Ian were the same age, shared a similar background, and became good friends. What Ian didn't know about biochemistry, Paul would fill in, and Ian would be quick to answer any clinical questions posed by Paul. Trish and Caroline grew close, two expats living around the corner from each other and sharing adventures in their new adopted home.

The Frazers learnt to find their way around Melbourne quickly, firstly because they were walking everywhere, and secondly as a by-product of Ian's decision to join an after-hours locum service as a doctor. Sometimes, especially before the birth of their first child, Caroline would go along too, as navigator. The move was motivated by money and, with the bills stacking up, Ian made the decision to work three nights a week, from 7 p.m. until 1 a.m., and one day each weekend. It did help their money woes, but it also appealed to Ian's business instincts, and he loved learning about the crucial steps to making an enterprise grow. He was back building something again. He ran his time at the locum service as a business, capitalising on the same skills that had enabled him to launch a medical year book in his final year at The University of Edinburgh for which he'd organised commercial sponsors to pick up the cost. He liked to build on what already existed, but some of his student peers dismissed the idea that a commercial enterprise would sponsor a student magazine. Ian took the opposite view; he thought medical companies would welcome an association with senior medical students, and he was successful in luring enough sponsorship dollars to pay for the magazine's production.

Now in Melbourne, the decision to work after hours was both helping out the family budget and exposing him to a new type of business. That business acumen would mark some of his later decisions, differentiating him from scientists who believed their work should start and finish in the laboratory. But the locum work also had a down side that constantly worried Caroline. One Saturday morning, after answering a medical call for help, Ian was confronted by a man wielding an axe. It was the surprise that threw him off guard: he had never faced anything like it before. With the intervention of police, the patient ended up in psychiatric care, and Ian went on to his next patient, his confidence rocked.

Caroline's new-found contentment also took a battering with the sudden death of her father, who had a heart attack at the age of fifty-eight. It was an emotional time – the birth of her child in Melbourne and the death of her father back in Scotland – and she started to wonder whether Australia might be home now for more than two years. It was a change from the way she had been thinking since Ian was first offered the job. It was around this same time that Ian's work took a detour. He was still pondering the hepatitis B virus infection question. He started looking at men who had sex with men: many became infected with the hepatitis B virus, and he hoped they might provide an answer. Coincidentally, he found that many of these men also seemed to have a damaged immune system. It presented questions that he hadn't considered before, and he was desperate to find the answers and determine any concrete link. Mackay gave him as much latitude as he liked, and Ian threw himself into his work. This, along with his love of Melbourne, meant the decision to board a plane and return to the cold clime of Scotland was serially deferred, and then eventually dropped. Each day Australia seemed more like home and the perfect place to bring up children.

Life was good and predictable, with many blessings along the way. Their second child, Andrew, was born in May 1984, Ian's workload continued to grow, and Caroline continued to enjoy her new friendships. But there were hardships too.

In November 1984, Caroline was at home with her two babies – Jennifer and Andrew – with the radio news playing in the background. Most of the time the radio was like wallpaper, a pleasant presence that she enjoyed but didn't necessarily focus on. But on this day something about it made her stop in her tracks. A fatal accident had occurred south of Melbourne, it said, involving a visitor to Australia. Caroline went cold, a slow dread creeping in.

Paul and Trish and their newborn son, Mark, had taken visiting immunologist Bill Ford from Manchester University for a weekend drive down to Phillip Island. The car accident was nasty: Ford was killed instantly and Paul Andrews was rushed to intensive care, where he died several days later. Trish and her baby miraculously survived the mangled mess. Ian had lost his sister in a car accident. Now he had lost his dear friend too.

He went to say goodbye at his friend's hospital bed, his grief worsened by the arrival of Paul's family from the United Kingdom. Paul and Trish, like Ian and Caroline, were just starting off, creating a family, trying to make ends meet and make something of themselves. They each had their foot in the door of a wonderful future. Ian was devastated by Paul's death.

As a child, Ian had a remarkable ability to put things in little boxes in his brain. It stemmed from both a natural intelligence and a reluctance to show too much emotion. He had dealt with his sister's death by trying not to think about it, by filing it in one of those little boxes in his brain, and in the innocence of childhood he had managed that well. It was so much harder now as an adult, and he felt Paul's death strongly. Caroline had never seen him like this; he didn't say much, but she knew by the way he walked and talked that he felt the loss deeply. She also noticed how he threw himself into his work.

Seven

People were panicking, egged on by both the broadcast media and the press. THE BLACK PLAGUE OF THE EIGHTIES, screamed a 1983 headline in the *Medical Journal of Australia*: 'Perhaps we've needed a situation like this to show us what we have known all along – depravity kills.' MOSSIES COULD SPREAD AIDS, yelled a headline in the *Daily Mirror* in 1984.

The death of three babies in Queensland as a result of contaminated blood from an unsuspecting donor continued to feed the flame of community fear. At least the disease had been given a name by then: acquired immune deficiency syndrome, AIDS. But in the couple of years before that, the same dread had swept through surgeries and hospitals, with some pathologists refusing to perform autopsies on patients, and doctors at one practice sneaking sick young men through the back door of one hospital and into unused beds. In laboratories too, researchers wondered whether they were putting themselves at risk.

Ian Frazer had been intrigued by this mysterious new disease since 1981, when he popped into a presentation by visiting Nobel laureate Baruj Benacerraf. Benacerraf was out from the United States and told scientists at the institute of a new illness he hadn't seen before, which was surfacing in the gay communities of Boston and San Francisco. Something had gone horribly wrong with the immune systems of these young men, he told them, and everyone was puzzled by it. That stopped Ian Frazer. It was as though a light went on, illuminating areas of darkness in his own research. When Benacerraf rose to walk back to his hotel, Ian jumped up and followed him out the door. He needed to know more.

With colleagues, Ian had drawn together a large research cohort from across Melbourne's homosexual community. When many of them became chronically infected with the hepatitis B virus infection, they also showed up as having a damaged immune system. But until he heard Benacerraf's presentation, each line of reasoning had hit a stumbling block. When the visiting scientist mentioned what was happening in the United States, Ian thought he finally had his answer. Was he seeing the same disease – whatever it was – here in Melbourne, Australia? Almost one in three men in his big study had a badly damaged immune system, and some of them had had more than one hundred sexual partners a year.

Wild theories abounded. Some thought the disease that everyone was talking about might be E. coli, but others believed it was the same disease attacking populations of *Antechinus stuartii*, a small mouse-like animal: when males of the species got turned on they mated with dozens of females before collapsing and dying of immune exhaustion. Were gay men in Melbourne suffering the same fate, dying from immune exhaustion because they'd had too many sexual partners? The fear that had gripped the general community also spread along the benches inside medical laboratories.

Dr Basil Donovan was one of four general practitioners who left a Sydney sexually transmitted disease clinic to set up a new private clinic. Gay men made up fifty per cent of his patients, with the other half being female sex workers. Donovan and his colleagues knew early on that something dreadful was happening. Reports were filtering in from the United States, and what they were seeing there made this small group of doctors feel sick. They knew that many of their patients travelled to San Francisco and New York and had suffered so-called Hawaiian Syndrome: too sick to make the journey back to Australia in one go they were forced to stop off at the island. Donovan and his colleagues, like others in Sydney and Melbourne, also started seeing patients who were complaining of fatigue, weight loss, and diarrhoea. All of them were gay. Stories of gay spa parties in the United States reverberated around conservative medical circles, with fear striking some doctors, who decided it was time to quit.

Seeking to answer his own puzzle, Ian and his colleagues sent a batch of blood serum samples, taken from their male cohort in Melbourne, to the United States for testing. The first lot came back negative, showing that it wasn't a specific virus that had caused their lymphadenopathy. But later, a new diagnostic test was developed for a different virus. The same batch of blood serum samples was retested and, bingo, there was a strong correlation between the results of those in the United States and those in Ian's cohort. The young scientist had stumbled onto why some people who contracted hepatitis B could clear their bodies of it, but other people could not. Ian's relentless pursuit of an answer had led to a significant breakthrough and he and the team put together a paper showing serologically that there was an additional infection and that this disease was common in groups of homosexual men: almost one in three in the cohort was suffering from the disease that would later bear the title of HIV/ AIDS. Even before the paper was published, his research started to attract attention and word, like the disease, spread quickly. He walked out of his science lab to go home one afternoon and was confronted by a media pack. Ian had never been interviewed before and was taken unawares. He stammered his way through the answers and failed to put a lid on some of the wild theories being raised about the new disease and how it spread. He went home knowing that he had not done a good job. A lesson in life, he thought: unless he was in control of what he was going to say and how he was going to say it, he would not again talk to the media.

An AIDS service was soon set up at Royal Melbourne Hospital, under Ian Mackay, but the hysteria grew tentacles and spread across the nation. Ian Frazer had always taken precautions in dealing with any body fluids on the bench; it was a legacy of the training he'd received in the renal unit back in Scotland. But with uncertainty on how infectious the disease was and how it might be transferred, he went home and talked to Caroline about it. He wasn't scared, just cautious. They decided he should just get on with the job; Ian put his head down and worked harder.

His Melbourne cohort also had something else in common. They were afflicted with genital warts. These were caused by a group of viruses called the human papillomavirus. The warts were not the type you had as children, where old wives' tales would have you tie cotton around their base until they disappeared. Ian looked up as many textbooks as he could but couldn't find much on the immunology of genital warts. More questions needed answers. In a stroke of luck, at around this time he met Gabrielle Medley, who was running the Victorian Cytology Service and whose interests focused on a connection between the human papillomavirus and cervical cancer. Cytology is a branch of science that studies cells. The association between human papillomavirus and cervical cancer had been made by a German virologist Harald zur Hausen but remained contested in some circles. The idea that a virus could cause a human cancer was new and went against the grain of many in the science establishment, largely because it didn't fit with tradition.

Gabrielle suggested to Ian that they go back and look at the men in his study to confirm whether they had the papillomavirus. He investigated the cells from their anuses. Eureka: they found pre-cancerous cells there, particularly in the men who had suppressed immune systems. It might not have been an answer to all his questions, but pieces of the jigsaw were now coming together, with one clue leading to another. Didn't this mean, possibly, that another cancer – in this case anal cancer – could be caused by the same virus as the one suspected to be responsible for cervical cancer? Gabrielle's help had been crucial, and they set about writing up their findings of pre-cancerous lesions in immunosuppressed men for the respected medical journal *The Lancet*. It created a stir, as expected, because it didn't fit with centuries-old thinking that viruses didn't cause cancer. But it also meant that for the first time Ian Frazer was on the map, and this finding signalled a turning point in a career that was still young and largely anonymous.

Ian's real interest wasn't HIV; it was the human papillomavirus, or HPV. He wanted to build on his knowledge of it, experiment by experiment, and he became obsessed. As far as science went, HPV didn't hold much lure for many researchers and its field of knowledge had yet to be tapped. Across the world, only a small group of scientists had any in-depth understanding of the virus, and one of those was Margaret Stanley, who would later host Ian in her Cambridge laboratory on a sabbatical. But that was well down the track. Now, at a bench in the Walter and Eliza Hall Institute, Ian just wanted to soak up as much information as he could about HPV. He kept up his other projects too, those that had been assigned to him by Ian Mackay, as well as looking at the molecular cloning of an antigen. He was busy at work, and at home, where Caroline toiled with two young children and not a lot of cash.

The crucial link between HPV and anal pre-cancerous lesions had turned Ian's interests firmly to HPV, but, as that was happening, so were things more broadly at the institute. Talk kept surfacing of Ian Mackay's retiring. Nothing was said publicly, but that was the corridor talk. Mackay had employed Frazer, was his supervisor, and Frazer knew his appointment was largely tied in with him. To some in the lab, it was Frazer's friend Mathew Vadas who looked like the golden boy. Frazer wondered whether he might be without a job when Mackay retired. He was doing good work, getting noticed, but knew he should certainly go before there was any suggestion he was being pushed. That's how science worked sometimes: an employee was seen as tied to the person who employed them. Ian Mackay also wondered what Ian Frazer might do next and told the young researcher's father as much when he dropped in on a visit to Melbourne from Scotland. His father had asked whether his son was in the 'very top drawer'. Ian Mackay wasn't sure how to respond.

Ian Frazer started looking at other opportunities, and they began walking through the door. He briefly flirted with a job in Boston and took Caroline across for the interview but climbed back onto the plane knowing it was not right for him or his young family. He looked at another research position, in Western Australia, but decided against that as well. He lodged an application for two National Health and Medical Research Council grants – one to carry on his work on autoimmune liver disease, and the other on HPV – and then heard that Princess Alexandra Hospital in Brisbane was looking for a clinical immunologist.

Brisbane didn't hold the appeal of Melbourne as a city, but he decided to apply and, when granted an interview, he was surprised to find the other short-listed candidates were sitting around the same table. They were all vying publicly for the same job. Ian left knowing that he had been the best performer, and was not surprised when the job offer came through. He was more surprised when the research grants also came through, as he had been successful in getting both. That didn't stop some of his colleagues laughing as he left the science world in Melbourne for the back blocks of Queensland.

Australian research was centred around the science and medical facilities located in Sydney and Melbourne, and a move north to Queensland was considered unlikely to be a step up. But Ian had never cared much what people thought and never wavered in a decision, once he made it. On his last day at the institute, at the end of July 1985, he walked into the office of the man who had given him his ticket to Australia. They had a chat. Ian Mackay felt a tremendous sense of sadness. Their relationship had been a complex one. Mackay had been tough on the lad he had plucked from Edinburgh, and thought he'd done everything he could to help him along the way. But he wasn't sure how Ian would go from here. On the flip side, Ian liked his boss but didn't always agree with him. The skills he had acquired under Ian Mackay's supervision would help him now, as he set up his own laboratory. Neither man was a big talker; neither man really knew how the conversation should go. They shook hands and Ian Frazer walked down the long corridor to the lift. Mackay watched him go; he saw him turn around and wave. Mackay waved back, wondering what might become of the tall, gangly Scotsman.

Eight

Caroline Frazer was part amused and part embarrassed. Here was her husband, who towered over everyone, climbing in and out of the window of a little Mini. He could only just fit by manoeuvring himself, legs first, into the car they'd picked up for a pittance. The driver's door didn't open, so visitors would watch her husband climb in through the window and start the car. Not that it mattered to Ian Frazer; it was a steal at the price they'd paid and did the job of getting him to work each day.

Appointed senior lecturer in the School of Medicine at The University of Queensland, he finally had his own research laboratory. Not that anyone could call his new digs flash: he was housed in the basement of the dialysis building at the Princess Alexandra Hospital and it looked more like a cupboard than a state-of-the-art science space. In fact, they called it the broom closet. Ian knew, from the moment he had accepted the job, that the heavy workload he had taken on would ensure this lab became his second home. He was required to teach, run research, and conduct diagnostic tests for the hospital. But on day one he walked in as though he owned the place, unaware of the rumours that had filtered through staff rooms ahead of his arrival. Ian Frazer, so the rumour spread, had wanted to charge the job interview panel for his time. It wasn't anywhere near right; nothing like that had happened. But the story was told and retold, and everyone was looking out to meet Ian Frazer. Some were intrigued. But just like the unflattering sandals he wore to work in Scotland, or the broken Mini he arrived in each day, the latest waffle – even if true – wouldn't have bothered the young scientist. It wasn't that he didn't care what people thought; he just went about the job in his own way. He'd done it at school, often to the annoyance of his teachers. He'd done it as a young doctor. And not long after his arrival in Queensland, Ian took it upon himself to comment on the government's inability to deliver an AIDS service. While many medicos supported his thinking, it was a different thing to come out publicly and say it. Soon after, Ian found the health minister on the other end of his phone, threatening that he would be out of a job by Monday. Ian smiled; he wasn't employed by the government and knew he would be turning up to work on Monday.

His hard work was paying off, but luck had also been kind to Ian Frazer in Melbourne. It was an opportune time to work on HIV because he had been studying a cohort of men who had sex with other men. The fact that many of them were immunosuppressed patients had also given him the opportunity to look for HPV that might contribute to anal cancer. That had put him on the map, but now in his little Queensland laboratory, with hardly any resources and limited funds to do anything, he knew he had to think of a grand plan. He had to build a state-of-the-art laboratory, in terms of research, funding, and even bricks and mortar. And he was given enormous latitude from The University of Queensland to do just that. He started thinking like a businessman and developed a plan. He needed funds and, with both hands out, he started seeking them. He was indefatigable in applying himself to the task, and it wasn't long before he started getting good results. His research money came from the two grants he had won, but that was just a start; he needed a big injection of funds first, and then skilled staff to deliver research that would make a difference, not just to mice, but to men.

With Caroline in charge of making a home for the family in a rented house in Highland Terrace in the university suburb of St Lucia, Ian nutted out his vision in the same way a company chief would go about his business strategy. He worked away at his brief: HPV would take a big chunk of the research agenda because there was so much more to learn. But as the appointed clinical immunologist, he was also required to hold two or three outpatient clinics a week, seeing patients with everything from asthma to lupus. The clinical side focused on transplant immunology – tissue typing relating to kidney, liver, lung, heart, and bone marrow transplants. With his background in HIV, he was startled at the ignorance that shrouded any political or public discussion over HIV/AIDS in his new city. He wanted to bring to Brisbane the clinical research that he had been doing on HIV/AIDS in Melbourne, to set up a specialist service, but Joh Bjelke-Petersen's conservative government fought any decent discussion. Ian rolled up his sleeves and worked, even visiting gay bars and pubs to establish how underground the gay movement had become in response to the growing public antagonism over HIV/AIDS. The process made him more determined than ever to ensure that HIV testing could be done in a confidential clinical climate.

But he knew it had to be done publicly, with the government looking on.

He was fortunate that Noela Strachan headed the clinical side of his operation, but he knew he needed a world-class research assistant, and the money to fund that position. The Lions Kidney and Medical Research Foundation, won over by Ian's enthusiasm and sell job, came to the party quickly, and he sent out the feelers to see who he could attract to Brisbane.

Bob Tindle was working in the United Kingdom. He held a PhD from the Institute of Cancer Research at the University of London and, after postdoctoral research at the University of Adelaide, spent three years as a scientist at the Charles Darwin Research Station in the Galapagos Islands. After a fellowship at the Beatson Institute for Cancer Research in Glasgow, he worked in the biotechnology industry as director of research at Sera Lab. He was perfect. Ian wanted him, and told him that.

Bob Tindle was not just good on paper, but an expert in monoclonal antibodies, or antibodies that are the same because they are made from identical immune cells that are all clones of a particular parent cell. They had first been derived more than ten years earlier by a couple of researchers in the United Kingdom. Bob set out to make antibodies to a particular protein, called E7, of HPV type sixteen (HPV16). Proteins, which are needed to make the body function, are like bicycle chains, with each link in the chain an amino acid, chosen from a total set of twenty different amino acids. It was known that it was this E7 protein that was responsible for transforming cells, or making cancerous cells, giving rise to cervical cancer.

Ian knew he needed to know more about how HPV worked. It was well known that HPV was sexually transmitted and it wasn't that long ago that it was found to cause cervical cancer, but science was silent on how it caused cells to transform, what the physiology of it might be, and how it operated. Bob Tindle and Ian Frazer did a deal. Bob had wanted to bring his work on leukaemia into the lab; Ian wanted him to focus on HPV. Ian agreed to stop his work on autoimmune liver disease, started years earlier in Melbourne, if Bob agreed to focus on HPV. In Ian Frazer's new lab – one funded by the Lions Kidney and Medical Research Foundation – they worked away, and it wasn't long before the first two major papers would come out of the Frazer lab, one on the E7 protein of HPV16 and one on the E7 protein of HPV18. Ian and his laboratory climbed a couple of further rungs up the ladder of international HPV research.

With Noela Strachan running the clinical operation and Bob Tindle beavering away at his HPV research, Ian also took on his first students. Arriving each day with a packed lunch, courtesy of his wife, Caroline, he would go about his many tasks. He kept encouraging his staff and students to think differently. They were encouraged to read outside their specific interest area, and spend time looking at the broader picture of what they were trying to achieve. That's how Ian Frazer approached science, and he was trying to pass that on to his students. It was his first gig as boss, and he introduced regular parties, barbecues at his home, and dress-down Fridays. Morning tea each day became something of a religion and it wasn't because Ian liked to have a chat. In fact, some of his staff thought he was a bit socially awkward. He didn't like small talk, but he wanted them to talk to each other about their work and share ideas. Ian was a team player and he encouraged that in his lab too. He joined in, inspiring colleagues with stories of new techniques he had read or heard about. Linda Selvey, now deputy head of the school of public health at Curtin University, was Ian's first student and remembers him coming in full of beans over a technique now used all the time, but not heard of then. Called polymerase chain reaction, it allowed researchers to amplify little bits of DNA. Now commonly used for diagnosis, she remembers Ian detailing what its future would be, and he was spot on.

Frazer's ability to attract money was also new to many researchers, and the Lions Kidney and Medical Research Foundation poured money into the lab to guarantee that research could continue. Ian was thoughtful too, remembering staff birthdays and ensuring that his staff always received the credit for their work, which he believes he didn't receive when he left Melbourne and another researcher took over his projects. It had left a sour taste in his mouth – he'd even had a go at his former boss Ian Mackay – and it made him determined that if someone contributed to a project, they should be acknowledged.

David Whiteman, now an epidemiologist at the Queensland Institute of Medical Research, took a year out of medical school in 1987 to do a Bachelor of Medical Science and Ian gave him the glamorous job of looking at genital warts and the different types of HPV that were occurring in Brisbane patients with those warts. His project was almost complete at the end of his time in the lab, so Ian tied up the loose ends and submitted David's work to a conference in France. He even found funds for David to attend the conference and, discovering his student was set to travel to the United Kingdom with his girlfriend, Ian organised that they both stay with his parents in Scotland. Members of his close-knit team repaid Ian's generosity and trust by laughing at his jokes, even when they were a bit lame, giving him a copy of a new CD they thought might be to his liking, and working hard in the lab.

At home, Caroline worked around the clock. Their third child, Callum, was born on 16 November 1985, and after renting for six months they finally sold their apartment in Scotland and threw the proceeds into the house next door in Highland Terrace. Ian was travelling and working all hours, and sometimes Caroline thought it was even harder when he came home. She and her three little children would establish a nice routine, with the house running well, and Ian would arrive back from some conference and mess it up. Mealtimes would be thrown into disarray, and she'd have to spend the next week working on rebuilding the schedule. Caroline also learnt not to rely on Ian, asking another father to pick up Jennifer after she had suffered a fall on a school camp, and even coaxing her, on another occasion, to go next door to seek help after Caroline sliced her finger while cutting a pumpkin.

But when Ian was home, he jumped at the chance to help, changing nappies and bathing the babies. And Caroline was thankful that he loved to cook, especially *boîte au chocolat* and their children's birthday cakes. He prided himself on the birthday cakes; they were never plain and Jennifer, Andrew, and Callum were treated to robots and fire engines and rockets and ships, all made and iced by Ian. His mother, Marion, was a wonderful cook and he loved starting from scratch just as she always did. It was a bit like building, or a science experiment, adding a bit of this and a bit of that and finding out the consequences. The legacy of that interest lies in the host of Frazer family recipes, where scribblings down the margin show how Ian would modify them to make the end product better.

Within a couple of months of settling in Queensland's south-east, both Ian and Caroline had found a rhythm and, after going along to an investment seminar, they bought a small timeshare unit at Tangalooma, where they planned to escape to each January for a real family holiday. There at the beach, body surfing, four-wheel driving and fishing, their children loved it. They were as Australian as you could get.

In 1988 they broke their traditional holiday in Tangalooma to make their citizenship official. Ian was on call at the time and could give advice by phone or quickly return by seaplane, if required, so skipping from Tangalooma back to the mainland was not too difficult. On the day they were to become Australian citizens they woke to a sapphire blue sky and perfect waters. They didn't want to miss a moment, spending the morning on the beach with their children. They waited until the last minute before packing for the seaplane back to Brisbane for the afternoon ceremony at Brisbane's City Hall. As they were packing, the perfect skies turned grey and then black, the waves grew in stature and the children began to panic, refusing to board the boat to get to the seaplane. Carrying them on, Ian and Caroline watched as their luggage fell around the boat. Andrew started screaming. Trying to console him, they talked about what they'd be doing in a couple of hours – becoming Australian.

It wasn't a tough gig; they weren't even required to give up their British citizenship. But it had been touch and go as to whether authorities would allow Ian to participate in the ceremony that afternoon. A prerequisite required that the applicant needed to be in Australia for a continuous set number of days, but Ian's heavy travel schedule meant he only met the rule by precisely twenty-four hours. That too was a motivating force when it came to the decision to call themselves Australian – it was so much easier to come and go if you were a citizen. The identity shift – from calling Scotland home to the sunny clime of Queensland – was gradual. They had intended to move to Melbourne for only two years. That then became four, before they decided to move to Brisbane and stay.

The Frazers made it back to Brisbane from Tangalooma, dropped their children off with friends, and took a seat in front of Lord Mayor Sallyanne Atkinson. The Scottish couple, in the crowd of hundreds, were anonymous, and didn't earn a second glance from others or the media. Ian wore his Marks and Spencer suit, bought for his first job interview twelve years earlier, and for the first time in their lives they stood and swore allegiance to the Queen. After a cup of tea, they picked up their children and returned to their St Lucia home as new Australians.

In the same year, Ian received his Doctor of Medicine qualification, but his real aim remained HPV. Bob Tindle continued to be his right-hand man, trying to understand the immune response in patients infected with HPV, and thereby how the body got rid of it. That was the goal then, not a vaccine. So much was unknown about the longevity of the virus and even how common it was. Did everyone with HPV get cervical cancer? How many strains of HPV were there? How many were dangerous? It was hard finding the answers, especially because they were experimenting on mice, not humans. Mice could not contract the virus because it was human specific – it was human papillomavirus, not mouse papillomavirus. Ian had to make transgenic mice to get to the next step, and the best way to learn was from others. He picked up his family and moved, on sabbatical, to Cambridge University.

Nine

In July 1989, Ian Frazer walked into Margaret Stanley's lab at Cambridge University, his home for the next few months. The university was founded in 1209 and was highly respected around the world. Margaret herself was an international leader in papillomavirus, and Ian had arrived with a purpose: to learn new techniques to make a mouse transgenic for human papillomavirus proteins. This would help him advance his own research into the immunology of mice. The molecular biology revolution had started years earlier, but the research to come up with a way of putting genes into cells so that the proteins could be expressed had not yielded any practical results. Ian wanted to study the natural immune response to the papillomavirus in humans, and he needed an animal model to do that.

Stanley's lab was stationed next door to the one run by Lionel Crawford from the Imperial Cancer Research Fund. Crawford's was better kitted out, so Ian would often venture next door to snare equipment, like the disposable pipettes he needed for his own research. It was here that he met Xiao Yi Sun who was working in Crawford's lab alongside her husband, Jian Zhou. The two Chinese researchers made ideal partners inside and outside the laboratory. Inside, Jian was the creative one, full of big ideas and possibilities. Xiao Yi was more organised and practical. He winged it; she kept a diary, working her way through tasks methodically, never not finishing a project. Jian would throw her a look and she would know what he wanted. Some people even commented that it was like having one person, but two bodies, in the lab. Xiao Yi was more outspoken than her husband, and perhaps not as patient. She watched the tall Scotsman from Margaret Stanley's lab come in and help himself to the resources in Crawford's lab. She stayed quiet, but after half a dozen times she couldn't help herself, and spoke up. 'Would you like to use the washable one instead of the disposable one?' she asked, referring to the pipettes Ian was taking. 'Thanks,' Ian said, and he took it. That conversation started a team and a friendship that would later dominate HPV research worldwide, and lead to a vaccine that could prevent the virus that causes cervical cancer.

Ian had been watching the Chinese husband and wife team next door in Crawford's lab. They didn't seem to go home, working day and night. But Ian knew they were there at all hours, because he was too. Caroline and the children had gone to Scotland to see Caroline's mother, and he took that opportunity to work as much as he could. Every time he walked into Margaret's lab, Xiao Yi and Jian Zhou were at the bench in the lab next door, quietly working away. Sharing the same tea room, and some of Crawford's resources, an easy conversation flowed, and soon they realised they all shared the same passion: insatiable curiosity about and a determination to understand HPV and its consequences. Ian learnt that Jian Zhou had earned his Bachelor of Medicine, Bachelor of Surgery at Wenzhou

Medical College, a masters at Zhejiang Medical University, a PhD at Henan Medical University, and had been a postdoctoral training fellow at Beijing Medical University in China. But it was his bench skill that impressed Ian.

Jian Zhou knew about viruses. His interest in HPV had begun with his study of the papillomavirus and oesophageal cancer, and he had spent years learning techniques for putting viruses into cells and looking at immune responses. The Chinese virologist was studying the behaviour and the characteristics of the HPV, desperate to find out how these viruses caused cancer. He needed to know how you could detect they were there and then how you might model the process of the cancer-causing virus. He didn't leave anything to chance and began cloning the whole HPV genome in a bid to make an artificial virus. It wasn't easy, but his benchwork was meticulous, matching his intellectual skill.

Ian Frazer watched from close quarters, impressed. The method of cloning bits of genes was primitive, and Jian stood out in his use of recombinant DNA technology, or technology that allowed DNA to be produced artificially. To the Scottish-born Australian who was working on how the human body responded to HPV, Jian's approach was more useful than making a transgenic animal, one in which there had been a deliberate modification of its genome. Like all scientists with experience in this field Ian knew that if he could make a fake HPV, he could infect cells with it and trick the immune system into responding as though it had been infected by the real virus. Creating a fake virus was the crucial step in creating a vaccine. Every scientist working in the field knew that, and across the world men and women sat in labs pondering how to make something that looked like HPV. This was the challenge.

The synergy of their work matched their personalities and,

despite the English conversation being stilted and Jian never touching alcohol, they would venture off with colleagues to the pub each Friday night after work. Conversation between the two tall, lanky researchers would almost always turn to HPV. Their similarities later struck many of their colleagues: as boys, both scientists had lived in a world of radios and broken television sets, and, driven by the need to build things, their work ethic fatigued many of their co-workers, who noted the trancelike state they could disappear into at the lab bench. They could sit there for hours, not hearing the talk around them. Outside the lab, their interests were similar too. Both loved cooking at home; just as Ian would experiment in the kitchen, Jian was the chief cook in his partnership, surprising his family with extravagant dishes he would spend hours preparing. On occasion, they both lacked tact too, as evidenced by Jian's visit to Crawford's farmhouse in Suffolk one weekend when he was served a traditional English pudding. 'I don't like it,' he announced to a stunned table.

Ian would later object to the colour of a traditional Scottish clootie dumpling he was gifted during a taping of Andrew Denton's show, *Enough Rope*, for the ABC in Australia. Ian Frazer and Jian Zhou both married gregarious, sporty women after falling in love early, women who matched their quick wit but were happy to support their husbands' busy careers.

Caroline loved Cambridge, and in many ways the family's trip back to the United Kingdom was her first tangible test of where she really wanted to call home. Of course, she had made the commitment to Australia the year before, taking out citizenship, and she was raising their young brood as Australians. But she had not spent any time in her homeland since boarding the plane with her young husband many years before, and she wondered how she would feel once she landed.

After spending eight weeks with her mother in Scotland, she and the children moved into a temporary home on the outskirts of Cambridge. Ian was travelling less, and she got to see him more. The children loved their new home, and, having all learnt to ride bikes – except Callum, who was only three – the family would cycle everywhere. Ian would lead from the front, with Callum on the back of Caroline's bike at the other end. Together the young family would explore the university town, eighty kilometres north of London. Sometimes with the children tucked into bed and in the care of a sitter, Caroline and Ian would dine out, always stopping at Margaret's lab on the way home so Ian could check something or other. But he never really brought work home.

Caroline knew her husband was working on HPV, and that a vaccine would be his eureka, but his comments about work were more of frustration: this had not worked, or that had not worked. Caroline let him talk and she listened. She had given up her own promising career years earlier to support her husband, and their children remained her priority. She loved that in Cambridge the whole family seemed to be laughing and learning along the way. Their second child, Andrew, started school there, and Callum joined the kindergarten ranks, providing avenues for Caroline to meet a host of different mothers, who became friends.

It was in Cambridge that Ian introduced Caroline to Xiao Yi and Jian Zhou, bringing them home to their cottage one afternoon for a barbecue. Xiao Yi was polite to Caroline but soon plonked herself on the floor with the three Frazer children. She sat with them, laughing and watching chestnuts roasting. She listened to the children's stories, and Caroline couldn't miss the look in Xiao Yi's eyes. She could see what it meant in an instant. Ian had told Caroline that the couple had a young son back in

China, but she was unaware of the details. Caroline could see how much Xiao Yi missed her little boy. She couldn't imagine being apart from her three children and wondered how Xiao Yi did it, day after day, month after month. But Caroline could also see Xiao Yi's passion for her work, and the pride she took in being her husband's assistant; and, over barbecued steaks and salad, the three scientists talked shop, each matching the others' insights. They all knew that across the world many researchers were working on similar projects, and, in a winner-take-all race, there would be no second prizes.

Nearing the end of 1989, it seemed as though Jian Zhou would be taken out of the race. Xiao Yi says he had received a letter from his postdoctoral supervisor, Naiheng Zhang, which he considered carefully. Naiheng told Jian that information didn't stop at the border, and that was the same for scientific research. Things had changed in China, she said, and money was drying up. His research could be done anywhere in the world. It signalled to Jian that his former supervisor thought that he could be on par with other international researchers.

The turmoil of the Tiananmen Square protests and its aftermath had changed so many things. Their son remained in China, and authorities refused to grant a passport for him to join them in Cambridge. It left them reeling. Perhaps their extraordinary good fortune had come to an end? When Xiao Yi went to bed each night, her silent tears would dampen her pillow. She just wanted to see her son, to hold him and remember what he smelt like. She didn't care where she lived as long as her son and her husband were both by her side. Was that too much to ask? Her trip to Cambridge had been planned as a short working visit, motivated by the invitation to advance her skills and see her husband. She was grateful for that, but now it looked like she was being forced to choose between the two males she loved more than anyone else in the world.

Jian tried to appear more stoic than his wife, but he felt the same. He started to believe that he had done the wrong thing by his family and was saddened that his own country now placed him in this position. He had always been very careful to acknowledge his Chinese education as the beginning of his fortunes and the pathway to all his successes. He didn't do it because it was politic; he did it because it was true. He had been gifted a good education under mentors he continued to call giants, and he wanted to repay those favours too. He looked for opportunities to do that.

One such case in point was the use of caesium chloride, a very expensive alkaline earth metal that can be used in laboratories. In China it was recycled, but not in Cambridge, where it was thrown out. That offended Jian's sensibilities. He wanted to send it back to China, purified. Xiao Yi was horrified. She thought it would reflect badly on them, and says now that she asked Jian not to seek Crawford's advice. Jian would not change his mind. So Lionel Crawford, who says Jian was always alert to helping researchers back in China, listened to the idea, patted him on the shoulder, and acquiesced. He made available a small room where Jian could store materials and old research instruments, clean them and donate them back to China. That conscience, along with his tremendous intelligence and work ethic, had impressed Lionel Crawford from the start.

Jian's drive also motivated his co-workers: Crawford would only have to mention a project as a thought bubble and Jian would start working on it. Within days, he would report back to his boss with the amassed results of the preliminary experiment and a complete plan for the proposal. And he could do it in a way that didn't offend anyone. Everyone liked Jian, seeing in him a good and quick judge of character who never bad-mouthed anyone. His colleagues laughed good-naturedly at his efforts to perfect English too: 'dodgy' became his favourite word.

Now, faced with the end of his time at Cambridge and with nowhere to go, Jian sat and thought. He knew every problem in his research could be solved, and he had learnt as a child that the way forward was rarely by retracing your steps. Perhaps there was a third country that would accept him and his wife and, even more importantly, their little son. He needed to build his career, and his family. These were the two pillars of success that his life revolved around.

Jian began his search for a new job in a new place. The CSIRO in Sydney wanted him and made an offer, but the position would have prevented him from focusing on his pet topic, HPV. Ian was also trying to help solve the problem for his colleague and friend, and provided Jian with Australian immigration information. Ian knew that Jian had skills he needed back in his lab in Brisbane. He knew both Jian and Xiao Yi would be hardworking and a great asset. He also knew his budget would allow him to employ both Chinese researchers.

He put it to Jian, who listened to the offer, barely able to conceal his smile. While Ian admired his colleague's bench skills, and knew how valuable he would be to the work back at home, Jian had also learnt much from the Scotsman, whose entrepreneurial mind impressed him. Ian could draw strands of information together to build a plan in a way Jian had not seen before. And he had witnessed Ian Frazer around his three children and knew that the Scotsman understood the heartache that he and Xiao Yi were suffering, without their son by their side. Their son would be part of the deal in Australia, where Brisbane would be their new home.

Ian Frazer ended his sabbatical, and he and Caroline packed up their family for a Christmas in Scotland, Ian knowing he had just made a crucial decision to advance his HPV work. Cambridge had delivered both the knowledge he'd sought and new research partners who would help the research already underway in his Brisbane lab. He also knew he was doing the right thing for this young Chinese family lost between countries, and he felt good about it.

A few weeks later, the Frazer clan landed at Brisbane airport. Caroline looked out the window and two words came to mind. 'We're home.' She might have lived in two Australian cities and become a citizen, but now she really knew. Cambridge had been a test. By the looks on the faces of their children, they all felt they were home as well. It was the beginning of 1990, and life was starting to deliver all it had promised. For Jian Zhou and Xiao Yi too, Brisbane would soon be their home. They started reading everything they could find on Australia, and dared to dream that soon they would be united once again as a family.

Ten

Jian Zhou, like Ian Frazer, was always going to succeed. His mother knew it on the day a neighbour showed him a combination lock and dared him to open it. Jian went home and sat in his bedroom, nutting out the various combinations. Then, each afternoon after school, he would race to his neighbour's home and grab the lock. Hour after hour, day after day, he would fiddle with the numbers, determined to break the combination. Then one day it opened and he carried it home proudly, the prize for the insatiable curiosity and unflinching determination that would characterise his life.

Jian Zhou matters in Ian Frazer's story in the same way fireworks matter on New Year's Eve. Their meeting at Cambridge University created the team that would be written into the history of science. They were scientists to the core: experts at the bench, working up to eighteen hours a day in a bid to crack the code that would change the lives of women across the world. But it was what each offered the other that made all the difference, and without that collaboration the history of the vaccine that stops women getting cervical cancer might have been different.

Jian was born in Hangzhou, in China's Zhejiang Province, four years after Ian's birth in Glasgow, Scotland. Before Jian reached his teens, his parents were carted off to the countryside in the Cultural Revolution. He and his sister were forced to fend for themselves, developing the type of independence that Ian Frazer, a world away, would have loved. It had an enormous impact on Jian and would be a story he would retell often, a driving force behind his work ethic in the lab.

By the time his parents were allowed to return home, China's Cultural Revolution was in its final throes, and school leavers were being sent to work in country and mountain areas. This dashed Jian's hopes of becoming a university student. He was ordered first to Chun'an to work as a farmer, and then later worked carrying loads of fabric from one room to another in a factory in Hangzhou, and then manufacturing wireless equipment at another. It was here that he captured the attention of his bosses, who were intrigued by the way he could build radios and nine-inch television sets from spare parts. As a reward he earned eighty cents a day, where some of his peers were handed twenty dollars for a whole year's work. A few years earlier, it was Ian Frazer's first job in the German car factory that brought him similar attention from his bosses. On different sides of the world, each young man was intrigued by spare parts and what could be built with them, and each was earmarked by his employer as a future leader.

When the Cultural Revolution finally ended in China and the tertiary entrance exams for university were reinstated, it was not electronic engineering that captured Jian's interest. He'd won the biggest prize of all, he thought, when he won admission into the Wenzhou Medical College to study medicine. It had been his first choice. He was twenty years old and it was 1977.

As Ian and Caroline, newly married and madly in love, began to set up home in Edinburgh, Jian Zhou attracted the attention of fellow medical student Xiao Yi. She saw the tall student listening non-stop to his cassette recorder and reciting each little lesson on the tape 'English in 900 Sentences'. To others in his class, like Xiao Yi, the English world offered intrigue, but not much more. The Chinese doors to the outside world were still closed and most students were content with that. To outsiders, Xiao Yi and Jian might have had little in common. Jian was quiet and worthy. Xiao Yi was social and chatty and sporty, a student sports convenor who played basketball, volleyball, and ran, danced and sang. In many ways, she was a Chinese sister to Caroline Frazer, the gregarious, sporty student who considered herself an equal match to anyone. And just as Caroline was hell-bent on proving that she could learn to ski as well as Ian, Xiao Yi waged a similar competition with the man who had captured her heart. Success was important to both Jian and Xiao Yi. Xiao Yi was jealous of his cassette recorder and how it stole his time. Jian was captured by her ability to love life.

Romantic student relationships were banned during this period, and neither Jian nor Xiao Yi dared risk their university education. But they were normal young adults at an abnormal time. They wanted to hold hands but knew it meant expulsion, so it started slowly, with a big tin of biscuits Jian bought for Xiao Yi so she wouldn't be hungry after sport. His first love letter was on a scrap of paper pressed into her palm. After that they would meet weekly on the bank of a small creek just off the university campus. Xiao Yi revealed her secret love to a friend, and from that day Hongxin Fan became their go-between, ferrying notes between the two and acting as a decoy to authorities. At ten each night the big dormitory gates would lock and the two lovers would scramble over the brick fence to meet up, looking over their shoulders, and their date would end with promises of the next time they'd hold hands.

In their second summer break, the couple sat in the lotus garden by the West Lake in their hometown of Hangzhou. By day they'd read books and wander the maze of garden paths, and they'd stay late to watch the sun go to sleep each night. It was there that Xiao Yi heard Jian define another sort of success, one neither taught nor measured by academic merit. An elderly couple sat on a bench nearby, their grey hair shining in the sunlight. They were obviously in love. That's success, Jian announced, to grow old together and still not be able to bear being apart. It would be a conversation, years down the track, that would haunt Xiao Yi.

As Ian toiled away in Melbourne, having taken the risk to move to Australia, Jian received a prestigious postgraduate offer to study at Zhejiang Medical University in Hangzhou. That in itself was a feat. Only one in every two hundred students was selected, and the academic who authored the national entrance exam believed Jian to be his most talented student. Xiao Yi, who was starting work as an ophthalmologist, was still waiting for her placement in a hospital, but they both knew it could be in the far west of China. Xiao Yi considered breaking their bond and sending her talented beau on to the success that he desperately sought and she believed was waiting for him. But he knew he couldn't do it without her. The compromise? He would finish his postgraduate training in two years and join her, wherever she was, if that was what she wanted. He yearned for success, but it was second to the success he saw in the ageing couple on the West Lake who still held hands after decades.

As Ian started to make a name for himself in his adopted home of Australia, Jian made big professional inroads in China. He was uncompromising in his commitment to work, even arriving late on his wedding day, in June 1984, because he got carried away in the lab. The next morning when Xiao Yi turned over to smile at her new husband, his side of the bed was empty. Jian was already back in the lab, working. After gaining a master's degree from Zhejiang Medical University, Jian's next stop was a PhD in pathology from Henan Medical University, which involved a long separation from Xiao Yi, who remained in Hangzhou. He also spent some time in Beijing, as part of that PhD. His world revolved around Xiao Yi, his son, Zixi Zhou, who was born in 1986, and his PhD research on HPV. He lived on noodles and continued a practice he had started years earlier of rugging up, without shoes, so that he could work long hours without the risk that he would fall asleep. He grew thinner and thinner, and Xiao Yi became increasingly worried. His colleagues told her that Jian had spent several weeks in the lab preparing his PhD thesis, with packets of instant noodles his only lifeline. Now, years later, Xiao Yi says she thinks back to those conversations and wonders whether it was her job, as his wife, to teach him the importance of balance.

When Jian was awarded his PhD in 1988, it was reported by *People's Daily* and Central People's Broadcasting Station. His ticket to the West was a step closer. His goal, he told his wife, was to succeed both in career and family life. He wanted to make a difference in science, be a role model for his son, and to grow old with Xiao Yi. It would be his personal trifecta.

Jian's postdoctoral training was in the Biochemistry Department at Beijing Medical University, where he continued his work on HPV. Xiao Yi moved her work and her son to

Beijing too, so that the family could be together. But it wasn't long before Jian developed itchy feet again, and was offered a once-in-a-lifetime opportunity – the chance of a fellowship at Cambridge University under Lionel Crawford, an international HPV research pioneer. Crawford was the best in the business, Jian told his wife, and he wanted to train under him. Xiao Yi listened and then told her husband to follow his head; his heart would remain with her and their child back in China. They would be reunited soon enough, and the time he spent in Cambridge would advance both his work and his family.

Not long after, Jian became the first Chinese researcher accepted by Lionel Crawford at the Imperial Cancer Research Fund at Cambridge University. It was Crawford who had finally given Jian his ticket to the West, and, as he prepared to leave his family, the couple wondered what the next few months would hold. It was Jian's first international trip and neither of them knew what to expect. So Xiao Yi decided not to take any chances – she hid two kilograms of solid soy sauce in his luggage, just in case it was unavailable in a country like the United Kingdom. And then they used their entire savings, plus money they borrowed from a relative, to purchase Jian's airfare. When Jian Zhou arrived in Cambridge, in the autumn of 1988, he had five pounds left in his pocket. But that wouldn't dishearten him. He caught a train from Heathrow to Cambridge, desperate to join Crawford on the fourth level of the pathology building, and before long everyone would expect those laboratory lights to burn well into the night. Jian, with pictures of his wife and his son in his pocket, had come to the United Kingdom to work.

Back in Brisbane, Ian Frazer was planning a visit to Cambridge University too. He wanted to further his understanding of HPV, and had his eye on Margaret Stanley's lab, which was next door to the one Jian Zhou was now working in. Jian hadn't heard of Ian Frazer, and Ian hadn't heard of the Chinese scientist. But science doesn't start and stop at geographic boundaries, and both were plugging away at similar research; it wouldn't be long before the tall Scotsman would meet the tall Chinese man. And perhaps it was luck that they would come together, or destiny, maybe, if you believe in that, but their meeting in a lab at Cambridge University would signal the start of one of modern medical science's greatest pairings: a team that would go on to create the world's first vaccine against a cancer.

Xiao Yi's work is sometimes not acknowledged because of her willingness for Jian to take the limelight, and the credit. But she was highly considered too, and Lionel Crawford offered Xiao Yi an opportunity to see her husband. Eight months after Jian's arrival, Crawford invited Xiao Yi to join Jian in his laboratory, on a ten-week scholarship. Her job would be as Jian's assistant. Xiao Yi believed her husband needed her. And she also desperately wanted to see him. She wanted to check whether he was caring for himself, and stand by his side as his laboratory assistant.

Xiao Yi was giddy with excitement. It was only a short trip, so she left her young son in China with her mother-in-law, whose support had allowed Jian and Xiao Yi to continue their medical work once Zixi Zhou came along. Xiao Yi trusted her mother-in-law with her life; they now lived together in Hangzhou, and Jian's mother doted on her grandson. Xiao Yi kissed them both goodbye and looked forward to meeting her husband.

First she flew from Hangzhou to Beijing. It was on the eve of the Tiananmen Square protests, and China was on red alert. It was so different from the last time she and her husband were here, at Beijing Medical University. She struggled with what she saw. Martial law was put in place, and then transport closed down. The city was paralysed. Xiao Yi could hear the chants of the students in the unit where she was staying. 'Support the students,' they yelled, louder and louder. Xiao Yi walked down to Tiananmen Square with thousands of others. She had never seen anything like it. But her attention was on a flight in two days to the United Kingdom, and she readied for that.

The next morning, all transfers to the airport stopped; no cars or buses were available. Xiao Yi found herself stuck and separated from the two men she loved – her husband and her eighteen-month-old child. What should she do? Would it be easier to journey back home? No, she told herself, this was just a hurdle. After all, she had a passport and official permission to embark on this adventure, and she had promised Jian that she would be there. And she knew she was excited too: nothing would stop her missing that flight.

So with the help of her father, Xiao Yi used a bicycle and then her own two feet to travel the fifty kilometres to the airport. She finally arrived at the airport, but instead of relief she felt panic. What was happening in this city? She turned to her father for advice. What would happen if she couldn't get back, if war broke out, she asked. 'Don't worry,' her father said, 'everything will be fine. Go and visit your husband – your child is in good hands.'

With a ticket booked for her return journey, Xiao Yi arrived in Cambridge as the Tiananmen Square massacre erupted. But she was now with Jian, and she saw no reason why they couldn't return home when they were ready.

Eleven

Jian and Xiao Yi were out walking the suburban streets of Jindalee in Brisbane's west. Life was good, with their little boy tucked into bed and Jian's mother looking over him. They talked about that day, several months earlier, when their son, Zixi – who later changed his name to Andreas – had come back into their lives. It still took Xiao Yi's breath away: the memory of arriving at Brisbane airport early, and scared. They had sent frequent photographs to Andreas so that he would know them. But what if now, after all this time apart, their own son did not recognise them or want to wrap his arms around them? Racked with nerves, the arrival time of Andreas's plane came and went. Jian and Xiao Yi stood in the middle of the arrival lounge at Brisbane International Airport. They checked the flight details; they had it written down correctly. Perhaps their son had been stolen, Xiao Yi thought with dread. Passengers picked up their bags and left. Families and friends greeted each other with big smiles. Xiao Yi burst out crying. Jian knew there had to be a plausible explanation and pleaded with airport staff to investigate. The explanation was simple: snow in Shanghai had forced Andreas's plane to Hong Kong and he would be arriving soon on another plane with his grandmother, who would also live in Brisbane with them. They waited for hours, playing over and over in their minds how the reunion might unfold. And then it was time. Andreas, still just three years old, walked off the plane holding his grandmother's hand. Tentatively, Jian and Xiao Yi walked towards him. They didn't want to frighten him. And then their toddler started to run, and so did Jian and Xiao Yi. 'Ju Ren Ba Ba [giant daddy],' Andreas squealed. Andreas, obviously taken with his father's tall figure, leapt into Jian's arms, and they all sobbed.

Now, six months later, Australia was truly home. Ian had welcomed them at work and passed on as much information about their new country as possible. But they also heard 'home' in the birds that visited the trees along the streets of Jindalee, smelt it in the jasmine, and saw it in the way their son embraced Australia from the first day. As Xiao Yi and Jian went to work with Ian each day, Jian's mother would dote on her young grandchild. She saw her job as supporting her son and daughter-in-law so they could put their minds to good use. The local news was all about the Fitzgerald Inquiry and the corrupt rot that had taken over chunks of the police force; and Paul Keating, the nation's treasurer, was signalling that Australia was recession-bound. But Jian and Xiao Yi felt privileged and rich, and their sense of belonging only sharpened as they made friends they could share it with.

Ian, Jian, and Xiao Yi were a close-knit team at work, and they were often there eighteen hours a day. Ian was the boss, but he worked the same hours and knew that Jian and Xiao Yi were driven by the need for success. To Ian it was clear: they had come here to build a better life, and that came through hard work. They arrived early each morning, went home late, and arrived back early the next day. They didn't mix much away from work with colleagues, but joined in functions for the lab. Jian was the archetypal scientist, Ian thought. He read widely, was focused on his benchwork, and was prepared to spend hours on one tiny step. Good jobs weren't easy to get, and young scientists were lean and hungry to be noticed. Ian knew he had chosen well. Inside and outside work, Jian would ask Ian advice: what about this car, is this a good suburb, how much should this cost? Jian wanted to soak up as much as he could, and he loved Western living.

Jian and Xiao Yi continued their fairytale romance, and no one remembers a harsh word ever passing between the two. Jian bought his wife a karaoke console for her birthday one year, and would then follow her to parties and to local Chinese community concerts as her personal DJ. On weekends, he initiated a neighbourhood rule: no one could come calling before lunchtime. Xiao Yi didn't sleep well during the week and her husband wanted her to catch up each weekend. So while Xiao Yi slept, Jian would take their son and visit the local markets, choosing vegetables, fruit, and groceries. Often, he would go the long way, so he could duck into the lab to check on his experiments.

Now, in February 1991, Jian considered his family life a success. But while Jian's career with Xiao Yi as his loyal assistant was progressing, the long hours were not drawing the successes they yearned for. Of course in retrospect, Jian's value to science can't be understated, and in his first four years in Australia, he authored eleven scientific papers – something Ian later labelled as a prodigious achievement for any biomedical research scientist. But in 1991, Jian's main goal was still eluding him: there was no doubting the potential to use immunotherapy against HPV, but without the technology to grow the virus in the lab, it was not possible to produce a vaccine.

Most viruses can be grown in the lab because the cell lines that are grown are 'permissive', which means that when a virus gets inside, all the machinery necessary for that cell to make lots of copies of the virus is present. HPV is different. It needs different cellular machinery during the successive stages of copying itself. In a person, the skin cell that has the necessary machinery to start the process changes naturally, as it moves from the bottom layer of the skin to the top layer, and, as it does so, the cellular machinery changes with it. The virus needs this change to complete the copying process. Ian and Jian had been unable to mimic those changes effectively in the lab.

There were many steps involved in getting from the concept of assembling the papillomavirus in the laboratory to actually producing one. For Ian, the aim was to produce infectious viruses, to study the immune response. One of the challenges was how to find small amounts of virus particles in amongst the experimental mixture that Jian was making in the lab by infecting cells with the viruses that instructed the cells to make the virus capsid proteins – L1 and L2.

'Jian and I discussed using a two-step technique I'd learnt in Melbourne to purify cell fractions by floating them on salt and sugar solutions. We tried this technique, and it worked technically, which was very pleasing.'

However, while the right protein (L1) was produced, it wasn't in the right place in the flotation mixture to be a virus particle. This puzzled Jian and Ian for some time, and they almost gave up trying to solve the problem, but rather than give up, they went, quite literally, back to the drawing board.

'We looked at the published genetic code encoding the protein we were interested in from the cancer causing papillomavirus (HPV16), and compared it with the published genetic code of viruses that were similar but did not cause cancer – there were not many of these at that time, and we weren't even sure that they were accurate.'

This comparison was done on scraps of paper, stuck on a wall, as the lab's primitive Amstrad computer was not up to the job. Ian and Jian noted that something was different about the virus they were working on. The logical start of the code of the L1 capsid protein of the cancer causing papillomavirus was different from that of the other viruses that were known at the time.

'We guessed that this might matter, and Jian made a new version of the gene that used the alternative starting position that was suggested by the other viruses.'

For the first time, they saw protein in the flotation mixture with the right density for a virus particle, though frustratingly, there was not enough to do anything with. Nevertheless, this minor change turned out in retrospect to be the absolutely critical step in producing the vaccine. With it, you could make virus-like particles. Without it, you couldn't.

Ian remembers thinking, when later faced with defending the patents protecting the vaccine: 'it was just one of many steps we took along the way – so minor that we didn't even note it as significant in the paper we eventually wrote – we just recorded that we'd done it.'

And yet, fifteen years later, it turned out to be the key to getting their patent granted.

One particularly balmy summer night in Jindalee, Jian and his wife were enjoying their regular nightly stroll. And when they started zigzagging back to their street, Jian stopped. 'Wait,' he said, before explaining his idea to Xiao Yi. She knew Jian had come up with out-of-the-box ideas many times before, and she was proud of her husband's tireless ingenuity. She also knew it was her job, as his assistant, to listen and take notes. So she listened as her husband thought out loud. They had two HPV16 proteins – late protein 1 (L1) and late protein 2 (L2) – at the point where they were well presented and purified. Could they replicate the protein shell of the virus, Jian wondered, but without the harmful insides, simply by combining them? Of course it wasn't that easy and involved genetic sequencing and molecular cloning techniques, but in non-science lingo, it was the bleeding obvious. Xiao Yi laughed. To her it seemed a bit like putting two cake ingredients into a blender, popping the mixture in the oven, and seeing what came out. 'How could it be possible?' she asked, almost dismissively. 'If it is that simple, someone would have done it decades ago.'

But Xiao Yi was a perfectionist and, as her husband's assistant, she made meticulous notes. When they returned home, she jotted down Jian's idea, climbed into bed, and didn't think much of it. Sometimes Jian's imagination was just too vivid, she thought. It couldn't work. She was reminded of another idea that he had laboured over for months. It hadn't worked either, and this latest idea was unlikely to be any different. The next day she went to work and didn't give the conversation another thought.

Life went on for two more weeks, when the couple found themselves again wandering the streets of Jindalee after an evening meal prepared by Jian's mother. It might have been a particular house or tree or smell, but Jian turned to Xiao Yi again and asked whether she had conducted the experiment he had talked about. Xiao Yi didn't roll her eyes. She would never do that. She was her husband's assistant, and he was adamant that they try this simple procedure. To satisfy her husband's curiosity, she decided to do it first thing the next morning. She would combine these two proteins under the conditions her husband had prescribed, and see what happened.

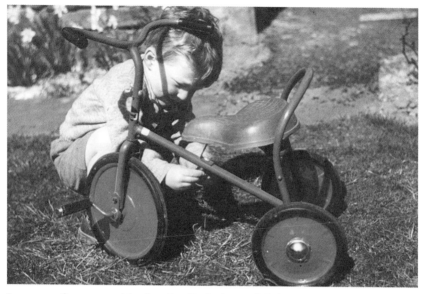

Ian, as a four-year-old, already displaying a life-long interest in problem-solving as he tinkers in the yard of his family's Edinburgh home.

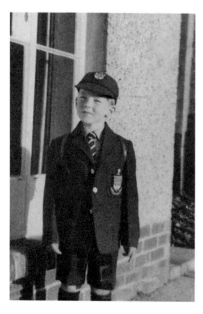

A five-year-old Ian ready for his first day at school at George Watson's College in Edinburgh.

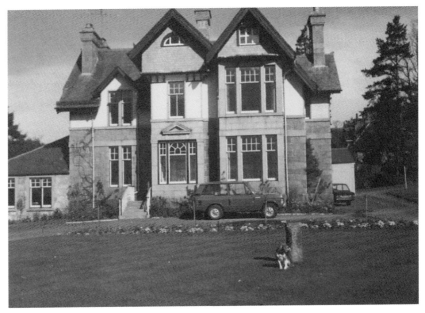

The Frazer family home, Murdan, where Ian grew up, just outside Aberdeen.

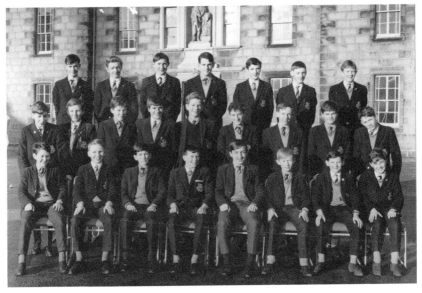

Ian, middle row and third from left, with his 1966-67 classmates at Robert Gordon's College in Aberdeen.

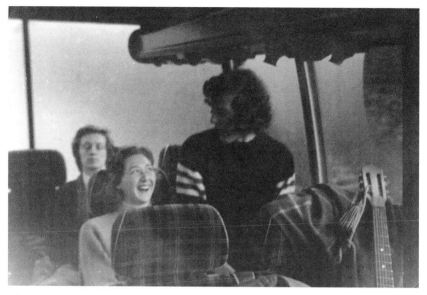

The weekend Caroline and Ian met in February 1973. The bus trip home from the university skiing trip was the beginning of a life-long romance.

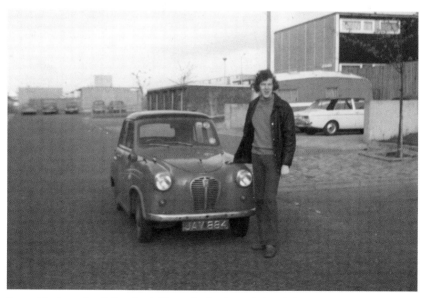

Ian with the prized Austin A30 car he built with his father. Caroline refused to travel in it, claiming she could see the road through the floor.

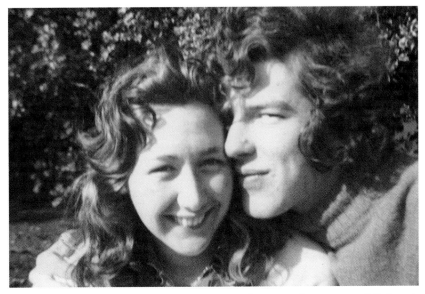

Ian and Caroline enjoying some time out between lectures at Edinburgh University, not long after they met in 1973.

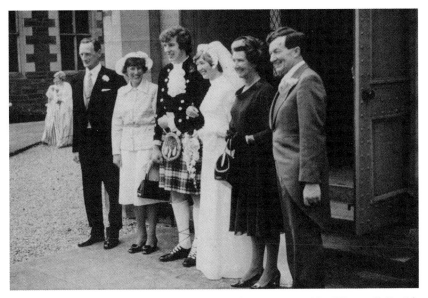

Ian and Caroline's wedding day on 23 July 1976, outside Kinnoull Parish Church in Perth, Scotland. Pictured from left: Caroline's father John, Ian's mother Marion, Ian and Caroline, Caroline's mother Lorna, and Sam Frazer, Ian's father.

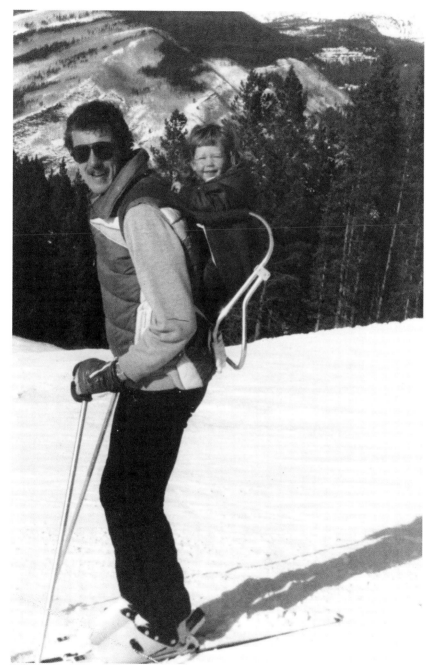

Ian and Jennifer atop the slopes in Vail, Colorado, USA, in early 1983.

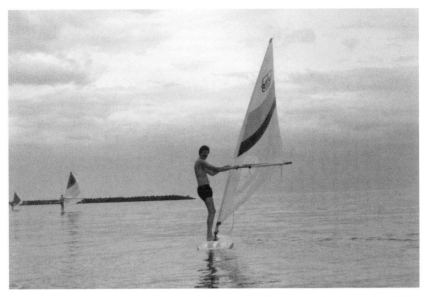

After work at Melbourne's Walter and Eliza Hall Institute in the early 1980s, Ian would often escape to windsurf on Port Phillip Bay.

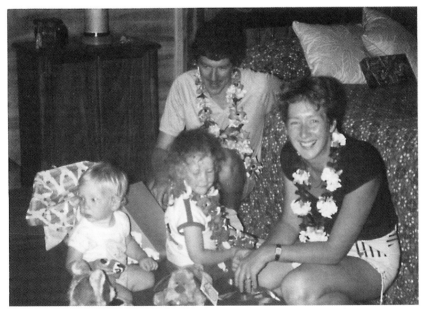

Ian, Caroline, Andrew and Jennifer on a family holiday on Big Island Hawaii, after visiting relatives in Scotland in May 1985.

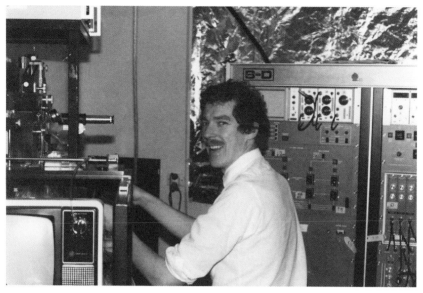

Ian at work in his Brisbane laboratory in 1986. Note the size of the computer equipment. (University of Queensland's Diamantina Institute)

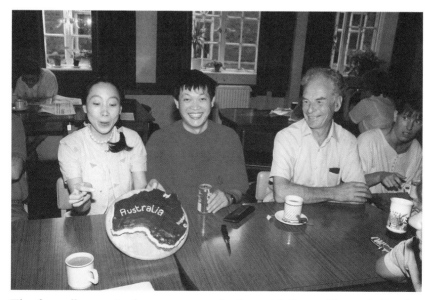

The farewell party in the tea room at the Imperial Cancer Research Fund at Cambridge University in August 1990. Xiao Yi and Jian are farewelled with an 'Australia' cake. Professor Lionel Crawford is sitting to Jian's left. (Xiao Yi Sun)

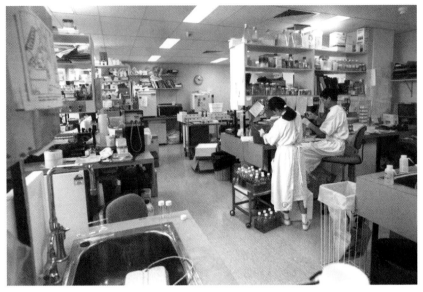

Xiao Yi and Jian at work inside Ian's lab, attached to Princess Alexandra Hospital. The couple had a reputation for working well into the night. (Xiao Yi Sun)

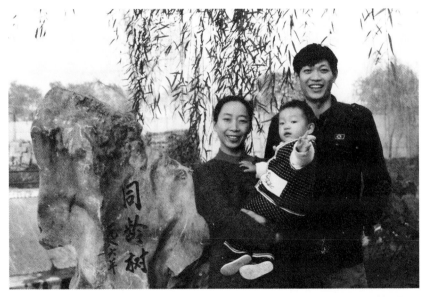

Xiao Yi, Jian and their son Zixi, standing in front of their apartment block in Hangzhou, China, in late 1987. The willow tree behind them was planted in the same year their son was born. (Xiao Yi Sun)

The next morning in Ian's Princess Alexandra Hospital laboratory, Xiao Yi conducted what she now jokingly calls the kindergarten experiment. With still hands, she put the two HPV proteins together, adding a bit of this and a bit of that. She did precisely what her husband had asked, so that she could tell him she had followed his instructions. She then made an appointment for Jian to have the experiment photographed by Deborah Stenzel, under the big transmission electron microscope at Queensland University of Technology. The microscope can magnify something up to a million times.

A microscope using light would not be able to pick up a virus-like particle – a transmission microscope uses electrons rather than light. Complex and expensive, the microscope was used on a fee-for-service basis, and Stenzel's value was in getting the best possible photograph.

And so this is what Jian Zhou had been doing in the first few months of 1991: he took a sample, got Stenzel to prepare it, and together they would lean over the monitor – which looked a bit like a television screen embedded in a table – to watch it. The first experiment hadn't produced any particles and nor had the next. Jian had his heart in his mouth every time he visited Stenzel's laboratory. Each new test was a step in the right direction, he would say, and Stenzel, used to working with scientists, thought she had never met anyone so enthusiastic about their work. Thirty-year-old Stenzel liked the young scientist too: he was always polite, always funny, and she enjoyed his visits. They'd huddle together in the dark in a room in the basement of the university's science faculty, with the small screen in front of them. First, Stenzel would get the microscope running and set the magnification low, around 2,500 times the actual size. A tiny sample droplet was then placed on the microscope's three-millimetre grid. Slowly Stenzel would ensure that she had the right density of sample. She'd scan around and then slowly, deliberately increase the magnification to 120,000 times the actual size. There were always false starts, with fragments of particles or big sheets of protein with knobbly bits that had not properly formed.

Stenzel was used to searching the tiny samples, looking at different areas, and sometimes Jian would offer his two cents' worth – let's have a look at that area or a closer look at what that might be. The resulting images were like an old black and white film. They were developed in a dark room and printed on photographic paper, and would throw up a better picture than the monitor. Jian would then pick up the prints a few days later and examine them in more detail.

Eventually, one day, and after many false starts, Jian finally cracked it. A developed photograph sat in front of him. He could see a virus-like particle – a VLP, or harmless virus casing that could be used to prompt the immune system to churn out antibodies. Jian, after hundreds of discussions with Ian Frazer and through the careful hands of his wife, had developed the shell of a virus without the infectious DNA inside it. It was a history-making moment: the creation of HPV-like particles using DNA recombination technology.

Xiao Yi recalls that Jian drove his second-hand silver Mitsubishi Magna straight back to the laboratory and then ran down the corridor to show his boss and mentor, Ian Frazer. Ian looked at the photographs, and then slowly looked back at his friend and colleague. He stared at the photographs again. He was used to seeing blank pictures, each new attempt promising so much and then not delivering.

They had so often imagined this moment, now it was difficult to fully comprehend. Here, in front of them, was a HPV VLP in black and white.

They'd done it, Jian said.

Back in Cambridge, Ian and Jian had discussed the expression of L1 and L2 proteins. Putting them together was always part of the plan – and putting them in the same expression vector was something they talked about often. Ian hadn't been sure whether it was technically possible. Jian made it happen.

Jian repeated that they'd made a VLP.

'No, Jian,' Ian said slowly. 'We've got a vaccine.'

Of course, Jian Zhou knew that the VLP would lead to a vaccine, and realised the impact of the discovery, but his boss's simple comment is crucial to understanding Ian Frazer. His mind had already begun to race to the next step. Where most people see trees, he saw the entire forest, with all its context and possibilities. This was how Ian's mind worked, growing up in the big house in Aberdeen, and now: each new step had to be built upon. He never stopped at the one just reached.

Sitting in Ian Frazer's office, Jian Zhou saw the VLP, the tiny particle he had been trying so hard to create, and felt immense pride. It had been a long journey across China, the United Kingdom, and now Australia. He packed up to go home for the night, telling his wife again how fortunate they had been. His boss had helped him achieve a success he could only dream of as a young child. Jian had delivered a code that had eluded researchers the world over. His persistence, in a game of trial and error, had won out. But he knew it was an equal partnership; from their joint decision to co-express L1 and L2, to Jian's idea of ranging the L1 sequence, to selecting the right method – a method Ian had brought to Brisbane. The technical skill of Xiao Yi shouldn't be underestimated here either. It had been a formidable team.

Ian, a cyclist, rode home thinking they were at the start of a race. He hadn't gone into HPV research with the dream of being rich. It was the search for an answer that had spurred him on for years, and now they had their first clue. But the next step would be harder; he knew that immediately they would have to find out whether the VLPs that Jian had seen under the electron microscope were able to generate an immune response, and whether it would resemble those seen in patients with HPV infection. This was really important – the response had to resemble the natural response so that it could neutralise the real virus if the VLPs were used as a vaccine.

Ian says now: 'Since we had such a small amount of material to immunise the mice, I knew this would be tricky.'

He also knew they needed a provisional patent to protect their intellectual property. Without that, it would be impossible to secure commercial interest to advance their benchwork to the clinic. It was fine for some scientists to talk about their work beginning and ending in the lab, but Ian didn't have a lot of time for that way of thinking. There was no point curing mice, he'd say: they were never grateful. To help humans, they needed a commercial partner. The benchwork was the brains behind a vaccine that could save the lives of millions; the brawn could only come from commercial partners prepared to invest billions of dollars to get the vaccine to market. A university couldn't afford that. A collaborative partnership was required to take their raw technology to the next level. They would start the next day.

What Ian didn't know, as he travelled across Brisbane to his St Lucia home, was that it would take another fourteen years – of funding fights, clinical trials, and complex international legal hearings – before the first teenage girl would be vaccinated against the virus that causes cervical cancer.

Twelve

Jacinta Stewart lay in hospital, her parents believing she was at death's door. She had lost twenty-five kilograms and two-thirds of her hair. The lymph nodes in her armpits were so big and red that she couldn't raise her arms. Her joints ached, and both arms were in splints so she could fall asleep each night. Jacinta was Anna and Ray's middle child, and they were at their wits' end on the day they carried her into Brisbane's Wesley Hospital to see Dr Jeffrey Forgan-Smith. Forgan-Smith was quietly spoken, even shy, but his reputation was excellent, and he knew something was dreadfully wrong from the start. Jacinta had been told repeatedly by a doctor that she was suffering from myalgic encephalomyelitis, a type of fatigue syndrome. But it had hung around and after several months, her condition worsened. In fact, she hadn't felt really well for three years, but in the past two weeks she couldn't even stomach food. Her parents witnessed the raging temperatures and the night sweats and asked that their twenty-five-year-old daughter be hospitalised; they were stunned when her GP advised against it, saying her immune system might not cope with the range of illnesses she could pick up in hospital. But now, seeing her in the arms of her parents, Forgan-Smith knew he had to act decisively.

Ninety per cent sure she had lymphoma cancer, he admitted her immediately to the Mater Private Hospital. She was frightened and bewildered and so were her parents. A biopsy of her lymph nodes was scheduled to support the diagnosis so that chemotherapy could begin immediately. The clock was ticking. Jacinta was extremely unwell, her parents were told, and medical intervention was necessary urgently, to save her life. The biopsy results came back. She did not have lymphoma cancer. But Anna and Ray's thrill at that diagnosis was shortlived when the reality that no one knew what was happening to their daughter hit home.

Ian Frazer took Forgan-Smith's call on Christmas Eve in 1990. They didn't know each other well, but Brisbane was a bit like a big country town and immunology was not a popular specialty. Ian Frazer stood out. Forgan-Smith knew he had gone into research, but he believed he might be able to call in a favour and seek his advice. He told Jacinta's parents. They had never heard of Ian Frazer, but were happy for anyone to be consulted if it could save their daughter's life. Jacinta remembers the tall doctor with the soothing Scottish lilt coming to see her. He had kind eyes and put his hand on her forehead the whole time he spoke. Ian could see the hope in the eyes of her parents too. They didn't care as much for his bedside manner; they were desperate to know what was wrong with their daughter and whether he could make her live.

Ian kept coming back to the raging rash on Jacinta's back. He ordered a skin biopsy, and the question was answered quickly. Jacinta Stewart had systemic lupus erythematosus, commonly known as lupus. High-dose steroids were prescribed and, by discharge, her patient record shows, she was walking around and eating. Her parents believed this Scotsman had delivered them a miracle.

But now, a few months later, it was millions of other young women on Ian's mind. What Jian had created in his laboratory was novel. The race had been on across the globe to create a virus-like particle, a VLP, because that was the path to a vaccination to stop HPV, which caused cervical cancer. The VLP would allow them to experiment in a way they had not been able to do previously. They had managed to create the shell of the virus, without the harmful DNA inside, which meant the human immune system could be tricked into thinking it was the real thing, and learn to repel it. But they were now only beginning. To develop a vaccine would take thousands of millions of dollars and a big commercial partner. The best way of attracting one of those was to own the intellectual property. Ian knew he had to establish a patent fast. Their results had to be written up and published for the world to see. A provisional patent on their discovery was crucial ahead of a big HPV conference to be held in Seattle in a few months' time.

Jian and Ian wrote up the academic paper, which detailed how they made the successful VLP and included the photographs taken by Deborah Stenzel. It was a rushed job, because it had to be, but they put down all the salient facts to ensure that others knew how they had achieved the VLP, and then they proudly sent it off to *Nature* magazine. It was the prestigious scientific journal where careers were made with a single publication. It carried weight in the international science and research communities and guaranteed that their research, if published, would be believed and cited by peers. Credit would also come straight back to its Brisbane creators, and The University of Queensland. But despite the significance of their finding, the lottery of editing contributions meant that their paper, called 'Expression of Vaccinia Recombinant HPV16 L1 and L2 ORF Proteins in Epithelial Cells is Sufficient for HPV Virion-like Particles', was rejected. *Nature* had said no to publishing their finding.

It was a setback, but a small one. It didn't have to be published in a particular magazine, but it needed to be published. They tried again, this time sending it to the journal *Virology*. With Jian Zhou as first author, along with his wife, Xiao Yi Sun, Deborah Stenzel and Ian Frazer, it was accepted. In the paper, Jian and Ian made clear what they had created and how it could be used. The virus-like particle could be applied in biochemistry research, the paper said, and 'provided a safe source for the vaccine development'. It was accepted in the same week that Ian and Jian were to present their findings to the international HPV community in Seattle. But before they boarded that plane, they needed one more thing in the bag: a provisional patent.

Robin Kelly was one of the few patent attorneys in Brisbane who knew what to do. He had previously worked with UniQuest, The University of Queensland's commercial arm, but this provisional patent application needed to be done urgently. UniQuest, at this time, was a nervous starter in any game that involved big money, after it had been sued by one of Clive Palmer's companies a couple of years earlier in a case alleging a breach of contract that was settled out of court.

Robin Kelly was called on to lodge the provisional patent application, which was essentially an ambit claim to a monopoly on creating the VLP and, if successful, provided exclusive use of it for twenty years. After twelve months, the provisional patent application progressed to an actual application. Ian gave Kelly the paper they sent to *Virology* as background to the application and, with staff from UniQuest, Kelly worked tirelessly and within days was walking down to the Australian Patent Office, with the fee of less than one hundred dollars. The patent was lodged just before Ian and Jian winged their way to the United States to reveal all to the world.

Ian and Jian were confident they had the trifecta needed to safeguard their finding: they had made the discovery that had eluded scientists around the world; filed a provisional patent; and their paper had been accepted for publication. At the conference, they performed a polished double act. Ian presented the findings, detailing their discovery and its consequences, crediting Jian, who sat in the audience before joining his boss on stage to answer the barrage of questions that came from across the room.

Ian opened his talk with a picture of an elephant with very large genital warts, and announced to the audience that there was great interest in studying papillomavirus assembly and immunology given the strong link between HPV infection and cervical cancer, as demonstrated by Harald zur Hausen and Lutz Gissmann. He went on to say that his lab had wanted to mimic HPVs for study, since there was no way of growing these naturally in the lab. He told scientists from across the globe that his team had made recombinant vaccinia viruses designed to express papillomavirus proteins. They had then used them to infect monkey cells in vitro and used these cells to look for protein expression. At that time, vaccinia virus was the only vector available for expressing protein in mammalian cells reliably. It was also the one that Jian had experience using. Protein expression proved they had got the experiment right – that they were making the right ingredients for a vaccine. Ian walked the audience through their experimentation, illustrated the VLP finding with photographs, and then declared that VLPs would become the basis of a vaccine to prevent HPV infection.

The response was electric, with some people hailing their discovery as the breakthrough the scientific community had been waiting for. But others were sceptical. Jian wondered whether his Chinese heritage was behind any of the scepticism. Others just wanted a copy of the elephant slide.

As the conference drew to a close, Harald zur Hausen took the stand. His stature in HPV research was unrivalled. Jian willed him to support their discovery, to give it the credence he knew it deserved. He held his breath as zur Hausen turned on the microphone. And then Jian grinned as the scientific giant backed their breakthrough, labelling it as significant in the search for a vaccine. The doubters had been put in their place. Jian was overjoyed but Ian wasn't surprised. He never doubted that what he and Jian had done was history making.

They boarded their flight back to Brisbane, believing that they had beaten the competition. For Ian, the reaction at the conference had proved that. What they had accomplished was made possible by a technology not widely accessible or known in the United States at that time. Ian and Jian contemplated the enormous workload that lay ahead; they had only made the first step in a long journey to a vaccine. They now needed to re-create the VLP, conduct tests on animals, find out more about HPV, and somehow finesse the technology to the stage where a big company would take a chance with it, hoping it would pay off. That would create a river of gold, but it was the discovery, not the money, that lured both of them.

What the two scientists were unaware of as they flew out of Seattle on 5 August 1991, was that some of those people in the audience who listened to their presentation would later claim that the Brisbane duo had been beaten to the punch, that the HPV VLP had not been an Australian invention.

Thirteen

Back at home, Ian took the ingredients he needed out of the fridge and put them on the bench. Slowly, he combined the flour, sugar and eggs. Each of his three children were either reading a book or outside playing. Caroline was reading too. He had the kitchen to himself and that's just how he liked it. He would start with a clean bench and, like a science experiment, he'd line up the ingredients. It certainly wasn't the only time he cooked, but making the children's birthday cakes had become a tri-annual ritual. He'd start by asking them what they wanted, and then set about building it. A rocket was easy: a few small cakes with the final one chiselled out to resemble the pointy space machine. A pool was fairly easy too: a big round cake with a slight dip in the middle and thick layers of icing to hide minor mistakes. This was especially important when one of his children requested a pirate ship. Ian didn't try and talk them out of their wishes; he considered it a challenge. Once the cake was made and modelled, he had to turn from builder into painter, and children can be hard markers. But each year that he was home for Jennifer's,

Andrew's and Callum's birthdays, he would make the cake and then sit back as the candles were lit, and appreciate what he'd built. The children loved it and so did Caroline. To Ian, it wasn't very different from what he did at work.

Cooking was a passion born during the time when he was grouse beating on the hills around Scotland and had to fend for himself. Of course his mother's penchant for making her own bread and using the ingredients in their big market garden played its role too. Now he had a list of favourites, headed by his *boîte au chocolat*. No one scoffed at his soufflé omelette or his steak in brandy cream sauce either. Later, he would keep a lemon tree on his back balcony and take the lemons and focus on a new signature dish – lemon meringue pie.

Whether it was a cake recipe or a new room for the home, Ian loved building. He built a concrete floor beneath their St Lucia home in the early 1990s, in case of flooding, and a retaining wall too, to keep the water out. He added a new laundry, and then a deck to enjoy the balmy Brisbane evenings. He was as comfortable with a soldering iron in the garage, as he was with a Bunsen burner in his lab, or the oven in their kitchen.

At work, he was building the science blocks to create a vaccine to prevent HPV, the virus that caused cervical cancer. At home, he was in the kitchen, building his next project: dessert. Just as the lemon meringue pie would become a family favourite to use the lemons amassing on their potted tree, his *boîte au chocolat* also started with a cookbook recipe, but his scribbled notations down the side heralded a better way of making it. He was building on someone else's work.

The family had a steady routine when Ian was out of town on work, which was more often than Caroline liked. Her meals would be simpler, and Caroline and her three children might tuck into a big tuna casserole, knowing that Ian didn't like tinned fish. It was a quick dinner solution in a busy household, where Caroline took primary responsibility for bringing up three active children.

Jennifer, Callum, and Andrew, all in primary school, had no idea what their father did, but they knew he was always busy. He worked at a hospital, and then often late into the night at home. On weekends, he would disappear into his little office, hidden under the stairs, and play with computers. He seemed important, but they weren't sure why. They did know that he could answer any question they posed. Routinely, around the kitchen table, they would sit asking questions, in awe at their father's quick responses. Why is the sky blue, Dad? What makes a sunset pink, Dad? Why do some people have blue eyes and others don't? Andrew watched him, vowing that one day he'd ask a question his father might not be able to answer. Ian loved their sense of inquiry, and often continued to explain the answer long after the children had lost interest. But any interest they did show was captured quickly and cultivated, in the same way his father had encouraged curiosity in him. Mirroring his own upbringing, Christmas stockings were filled with chemistry sets and CSIRO science club memberships, and reading was fostered from an early age, sometimes even involving an over-the-phone bedtime story from another country. Jennifer was reading *The Hobbit* by the age of nine and, soon after, *The Lord of the Rings* trilogy; she even surprised her year four teacher when she wanted to discuss the medical thriller *Coma* by Robin Cook. Science fiction lured Ian in from an early age, and he passed that down to his young children, along with the importance of good research skills. As primary school students, they were urged to look up definitions in a dictionary and search for answers in the big set of encyclopaedias they had been bought. Sometimes Ian would take them down the road to The University of Queensland and show them how to find something on the library card catalogue system. Life was about experience, he and Caroline believed, and with a limited budget they gave their children everything they could. Piano lessons from the age of five. Cheap seats at the opera when they were not much older, hoping they would grow to love Mozart and Verdi and Puccini as much as their parents.

On the weekend, Ian would sit on the sideline of their soccer matches, engrossed in his laptop, leaving the cheering to other parents. The Frazer children decided what sports they joined, and Ian wasn't interested in recording every touch of the ball. But when he could help, he did, and it was the local swimming club that benefited the most. Each Friday night, dozens of children would dive into the pool, racing against themselves in a bid to achieve a new personal best time. It was fun but chaotic and disorganised, and Ian decided he needed to fix it. He began building a basic computer program that could order races, times, and swimmers automatically. It meant that children could easily be ordered into the right races and the right lanes, and their times could be recorded correctly. It took a couple of meets for Ian to test and tweak it, but he then handed it over to the swimming club, along with a computer and printer. It changed Friday nights.

Ian would miss those nights as work increasingly took him away. During those times Caroline was Mum and Dad to their three youngsters, sometimes calling on the help of other parents. Caroline, as well as the children, looked forward to their annual holidays when Ian would down tools and become a full time dad. This had been their reason for the purchase of the time-share unit in Tangalooma in their first year in Brisbane, and each January they would head off for a week of swimming, surfing, and fishing. Ian would take to the sand in a four-wheel drive, thrilling his children, and then play computer games they believed he had bought as much for himself as for them. He would spend time teaching them board and card games too, particularly chess, whist, bridge, and mahjong, without the gambling. The kids knew their dad only ever lost when he let someone else win.

Family skiing trips took them further afield, to Perisher and Thredbo in Australia and eventually the United States and Europe; and, while they were no less fun, they were exhausting. Each morning, as the sun was rising, the Frazers would wake, eat, get dressed, and be ready to catch the first ski lift of the day. Hour after hour they would hurtle down slopes, Ian taking them higher and higher, creating a bigger and bigger adventure. The days passed quickly, and the Frazers usually skied back down the mountain after the last scheduled chairlift. The children would fall into a deep sleep, exhausted, unaware that other families broke up their daily skiing with shopping, reading, and even sleeping in.

The ski fields offered Ian the only real respite from the race that began the moment that he and Jian arrived home from the Seattle HPV conference. The world now knew that two scientists in a laboratory in Australia had created a HPV VLP, and every big pharmaceutical company now wanted a part of it and the vaccine it promised. Ian's phone did not stop.

The Commonwealth Serum Laboratories, which became CSL Limited, and incorporated in 1991, always had the inside running, thanks to a relationship Ian formed with CSL scientist Stirling Edwards a few years earlier. Back then, directors at CSL wanted to change its business direction, and it started to focus on opportunities for likely vaccines. Stirling, who had previously worked with cervical cancer, suggested HPV. He began to search for experts in the field, and was given the name of Ian Frazer. Stirling found him at the Princess Alexandra Hospital, and in mid-1990, a year before Jian and Ian could lay claim to creating history, he picked up the phone. A few others inside CSL didn't agree with Stirling's enthusiasm, still sceptical that a virus could cause a cancer, or, even if that were true, whether you could create a vaccine against it. Stirling wasn't put off and, six weeks later, Ian and Stirling met up at CSL's headquarters in Melbourne. Ian knew his laboratory could only grow with corporate research funding. An arrangement was quickly formed where CSL supplied Ian with resources on the understanding it got first dibs on his lab's early intellectual property. The arrangement led to a patent not relating to VLPs being lodged, and laid the groundwork for a more formal agreement the following year. With Ian Gust's appointment as research and development director at CSL, the company ramped up its support for Ian's lab. Ian Gust and Ian Frazer had known each other since they collaborated on a project years earlier in Melbourne, and Gust pushed hard to nurture the relationship between his organisation and the talented Brisbane scientist.

When Jian and Ian made the VLP breakthrough, Ian knew he and The University of Queensland couldn't take it much further. That frustrated him. When would medical science be seen as a bench-to-bedside discipline, he wondered. Ian vowed that one day he'd build a science facility where scientists could focus on medical breakthroughs that could be trialled under the same roof. But right now, their discovery needed a big pharmaceutical company to bankroll the science, launch trials and, if successful, develop an international manufacturing and distribution system. He knew he had to hand it over to someone else, and CSL was the best candidate.

It wasn't long before international companies were knocking on CSL's door. Inside laboratories around the world, scientists were trying to be the first to nail a vaccine. Others had also made VLPs, and big pharma was desperate to sew up deals to catch the revenue that would eventually flow. Of course, most companies were ruled out of the bidding because of the size of the project. Delivering a vaccine en masse to the United States required a billion-dollar commitment. Factories would need to be built, housing thousands of employees dedicated to the task over the years ahead. But that was down the track. First up, the intellectual property rights had to be traded. One of those to approach CSL was the big US company Merck & Co., which had a team of scientists working on HPV and a vaccine, but they needed help. They needed Ian and Jian's research.

Ian and Jian and their colleagues continued to work, trying each day to advance their knowledge of HPV. Why did it do this, and not that? Did it infect all people to the same degree? What made someone able to shed the virus, but not others? The research grew different tentacles, and two years after the VLP's discovery Ian and Jian made an infectious HPV in the laboratory for the first time. This was used to prompt immune responses in animals. Each step gave them a better understanding of HPV and its modus operandi.

Early in 1995, after long negotiations, CSL on-licensed Jian and Ian's work to Merck & Co. The deal meant that CSL had the rights to distribute any vaccine that was created in Australia and New Zealand, but Merck & Co. would be granted the global rights, including the most lucrative market – the United States. CSL would receive a big annual royalty payment back from Merck & Co., and would then pay royalties to UniQuest, The University of Queensland's commercial arm. That share alone would amount to millions of dollars, if the vaccine succeeded. Out of that, Jian and Ian would also receive a share.

It wasn't an easy negotiation, with each party looking out for its own interest. UniQuest boss David Evans sought help from an expert in the United States, Alex Scott. Alex, whose specialty was helping smaller companies raise money and license products, backed Evans for UniQuest, pushing for a better deal. His concern was that CSL was not sharing enough of what would come downstream in profits, and he suggested that UniQuest go back to the negotiating table. CSL was also pushing for the best deal with Merck & Co.

Ian looked on, believing that he and Jian were about to be dudded. The University of Queensland was in the process of changing its intellectual property policy. It had long been established that the inventor received a payment upfront, and nothing down the track, and that's what Jian and Ian had signed up to years earlier. But this was changing to a deal whereby they received a third of whatever the university collected in royalties.

Ian had held long talks with UniQuest boss David Evans about it; the new policy would value the inventor more and encourage research development. But Ian and Jian were eventually told they would not receive what they believed they had been promised: the university was holding them to the old written agreement. Ian had witnesses to the conversations, but nothing was in writing. He was miffed, and he told those running the university. At one stage he even threatened to go to the media. It dragged on and on, beyond the deal between UniQuest, CSL and Merck & Co., and became a sticking point over several years between the university and Ian. The HPV VLP had been a creation in his laboratory, under his guidance, and he believed the university should honour the verbal agreement. More than the money, Ian was furious that someone had reneged on a promise. Eventually, university chiefs realised the power that Ian Frazer and his science could wield for the university and formalised the new agreement, which still exists today. Royalties are divided equally each year between Ian Frazer and the estate of Jian Zhou, who died before the new deal was signed. Jian had an inkling he would be responsible for a vaccine that could save, over time, millions of women's lives, but never any proof.

The University of Queensland certainly didn't lose out in the deal it cut with CSL and Merck & Co. in 1995. All Ian Frazer's lab could offer, at that stage, was animal data that the potential vaccine had produced an immune response: mice had been vaccinated and the response suggested they were protected from the virus. It was well short of a vaccine, which would need scalability, a target market, and broad efficacy. It was a gamble for all the parties. But everyone knew that if a vaccine did result, they would all win.

By the time the international licensing deal was signed, Ian was well into planning an international papillomavirus conference on the Gold Coast. He had lobbied for it to be at Surfers Paradise, even calling on Harald zur Hausen, who had first recognised the connection between HPV and cervical cancer, to support the bid. And now, with the conference only a year away, Ian was stuck. Interest had flowed in from around the world, especially on the back of his and Jian's discovery, but now he needed money to make it work. Down payments were needed at venues, for social events, and to hold accommodation, and Ian's approach to both government and his own university had fallen on deaf ears. About thirty thousand dollars had been raised from corporate partners and the National Institutes of Health in the United States, because it wanted some of its students to attend. But he still needed over one hundred thousand dollars or the event would have to be cancelled.

He reconsidered the figures, and asked some suppliers to defer accounts. He had learnt, over the years, to ask for donations, and he was now putting that practice to good use. He then decided to take all bookings and registrations over the web. He used HTML language to make booking forms, at a time when this was unusual. He also gave discounts for 'early bird' registrations, something not offered previously for science conferences. And then, after talking to Caroline, he went cap in hand to the bank to ask for a loan; he borrowed $110,000 and took out a second mortgage on the family home. Three months later, with enough forward registrations, he was able to pay it back, and the international conference drew HPV experts from around the world.

But as they were gathering on a hot December day in 1996 on Queensland's Gold Coast to mark the fifteenth annual international papillomavirus conference, the United States Patent and Trademark Office was closing in on a decision that would turn the race to make a vaccine on its head. Within months it would declare something called an 'interference hearing' – an investigation to work out who deserved the patent. Ian and Jian's VLP discovery was being questioned from three different quarters, and the scene was set for a decade-long, multi-million-dollar legal brawl.

Fourteen

It was 2004, more than a decade after their 1991 VLP triumph, and Ian Frazer had just had the worst day of his life. The next day threatened to be no better. Caroline could see it, as she sat across the table from him in a small Washington restaurant. Ian had spent seven hours answering questions, trying to convince United States attorneys that he and Jian were the inventors of the HPV VLP. But their questions had been relentless. One after another. Hour after hour. Ian noticed in the afternoon how they started asking the same questions, but from different angles. His lawyers had warned him of that. But it seemed like a game, and he wasn't interested in playing. What made it worse were the rules attached to the hearing. He'd only been to court once, as an expert witness in a paternity hearing in Australia. This was entirely different: he couldn't refer to notes, his lawyers couldn't interrupt the questioner, he couldn't seek advice. He was on his own and hoped that his memory of what had happened years ago, when he first saw the photographs Jian had shown him of the VLP, was enough to get him through.

He'd worn his Marks and Spencer suit, which he'd owned now for more than twenty years, but usually reserved for upmarket work functions or awards ceremonies or even nights out with Caroline. Today, it had been a hearing to work out who first created the VLP, the crucial first step in developing a vaccine for cervical cancer. And in eleven hours, Ian knew he had to be back to face more questions. He wondered what they might be. He'd already been asked about every notation he had made, every work diary entry, and every conversation he'd had about VLPs, but the US attorneys continued to want more. They'd even asked for emails from 1991, which were on a computer that had been mothballed by The University of Queensland. But this hearing was worth a mint to The University of Queensland, and CSL had put no limit on the price of winning. His lawyers had ensured that the old computer was found and the hard disk retrieved. Someone was then paid to build a machine that could read the disk. A separate operating system was also built to ensure the software worked and the emails could be read.

Ian had no idea how much it all would have cost, but he found out later that the email everyone was looking for didn't hold the information needed. It was a measure of how serious this hearing was. He couldn't even talk to Caroline about the day he'd just had; he'd been warned about that, over and over.

During a light meal, and a single glass of wine, Ian and Caroline talked about their children and how, within forty-eight hours, they would be on a plane and winging their way back to Brisbane. Now, as he had many times before, Ian deeply missed his friend and colleague Jian, who had died in 1999, and taken with him some of the answers to the questions lawyers were now asking, including diary dates. Ian missed Jian personally as much as he did professionally; they had been a team, with the dream of creating the vaccine that would stop women contracting cervical cancer. After this day of questioning, the irony – of Jian losing his life early after spending his career trying to allow women to live longer – was not lost on Ian or Caroline. The Frazers finished their meal, their minds already back home.

Science never moves in a straight line, and the fifteen years after Ian and Jian first looked at photographs of the VLP showed that better than anything. There were fits and starts, regular u-turns, and constant obstacles as each new experiment raised yet another question. Every tiny step took time and patience. Experienced scientists accepted that, but it didn't take away from the frustration. Acknowledgement was part of the process: a finding had to be accepted, then published. Sometimes this took weeks and sometimes years, but eventually it would add a building block to the knowledge held by the scientific community. In labs across the world, people worked together, building up the blocks of knowledge, each using the work of other scientists, with the collective aim of making a difference. It was fiercely competitive, but few lost sight of the main aim.

The law is similar in some ways. Each new legal precedent adds to the way communities are run, but the wheels of justice can be painstakingly slow and complex. The big discovery in Ian's lab mixed science, the law and money. It had already added a building block to the world of immunology, but it was the financial spoils that needed to be nutted out, and whoever was declared the inventor would be rewarded handsomely.

The legal battle began in 1997 when the United States Patent and Trademark Office called the interference hearing. It wasn't as simple as granting Jian and Ian the patent in the United States, the Patent and Trademark Office said in its decision to launch the hearing, because they had received several other applications from scientists claiming to have beaten them to the punch. They believed that they, not The University of Queensland, should be declared the patent holders for the lucrative US market. The US patent system is filled with peculiarities to those outside it. It is based on the principle that the first to invent is not necessarily the first to lodge a patent, so even though Ian Frazer had been the first to lay claim to inventing the HPV VLP, other parties could lay the same claim. And that is exactly what happened to Ian and Jian, who lodged their patent in Australia in July 1991, and in the United States months later, as the law required.

Georgetown University filed a provisional patent in June 1992, the National Institutes of Health in September the same year, and Rochester University in March 1993. So while patent law in the rest of the world revolved around the first to file a patent, US patent examiners had to determine who was the first to invent the VLP. And that's why, in June 1997, the Patent and Trademark Office allowed United States attorneys to cross-examine other parties' witnesses. Was it Ian Frazer and Jian Zhou from Australia who were the first to invent, as well as lodge the patent? Or was it one of the other parties, all from the US, who had first created the crucial VLP?

Until 2007, that question would play out in court hearings. The prize, for the scientist, was international acclaim. The prize for those organisations behind them – the universities and the companies that had signed up to use their intellectual property – was a multi-million-dollar revenue stream. Everyone fronting these hearings understood that, and millions of dollars were spent to quash the other parties' claims. John Cox, the chief strategist for the Australian case, believed the lawyers for the other parties couldn't wait to get their hands on the Queensland scientists. They wouldn't come across as criminal lawyers; their bull terrier instincts would be hidden behind good manners and clever language. But a single error, after hours of questioning, could signal the end of the Australian case. The Australians just had to contradict themselves, or dispute something they had previously argued.

John was working with CSL's lawyer Peter Turvey, US attorney Beth Burrous, who had trained originally as a scientist, and a team of others. They knew they had a good case and had schooled Ian up on how to answer questions ahead of his 2004 appearance. They had prepared question after question, knowing anything could be asked of the Australian scientist, who understood the significance of the hearing, but would have preferred to have been back in his Brisbane laboratory, working with mice.

Ian had worked hard to prepare for the hearing, repeating time and again, what had happened and when. John liked this tall Scotsman. He, along with Jian Zhou, had invented the first HPV VLP and he felt the United States Patent and Trademark Office should recognise that. For Ian Frazer it was a question of ethics; so when he walked out of the hearing to go to dinner with Caroline, John Cox couldn't help but feel a bit nervous. Beth Burrous felt the same. She had told Ian to be clear in his answers, and to only answer the question asked.

Beth knew from experience that that was where things could become unstuck, and this hearing was unlike any other she had been involved in: it included hundreds of witnesses, many of them scientists. Each party had a pack of lawyers trying to make each other's witnesses slip up. Beth liked that part; she'd researched the case meticulously and enjoyed leading witnesses down a track. What was wrong with Ian's claims? Why wasn't the experiment by Ian and Jian valid? What was it missing? They'd answer, and then Beth would pounce.

'Why then,' she would ask, 'did you reference Jian and Ian's work in your own academic papers before this hearing began? Why did you feel compelled to write glowingly of what had been discovered in Ian Frazer's lab' – in this paper or that paper – 'and now you are rubbishing it?' It was the surprise on the faces of some of the witnesses she enjoyed most.

Ian Frazer's team thought his biggest competitor was the National Institutes of Health, and its lawyers used the argument that Jian could not have produced a proper VLP because he had used a prototype HPV16, L1 sequence, rather than genuine, or 'wild' protein. This was crucial because, they argued, if they had used prototype, they had not formed proper VLPs, an argument that, if successful, would destroy anything Ian had claimed prior to the day he lodged the patent in the United States – not Australia. The National Institutes of Health also worked to establish that a prototype HPV16 VLP had no practical use. Its claim was long and loud, and, while its admission that it, in its priority patent, had also used prototype – and not the real thing – in attempting to make VLPs would jeopardise its chance of winning, it would also end up sinking Ian Frazer and Jian Zhou's case.

Rochester University supported the National Institutes of Health, as did Georgetown University, but it also argued that it had invented something different from that of Ian Frazer. Hundreds and hundreds of witness statements were taken as the months passed, and then years. There were so many parties that at one stage lawyers were given strict time limits on how long they could question witnesses. At first it was the three US parties against Frazer. Along the way that changed and was replaced by six concurrent two-way hearings. It was a lawyers' picnic, as legal bills quickly ran into the millions. Similar hearings were gearing up in other jurisdictions, like Europe and Canada, but they became sideshows; the United States was the big market that would eventually reap billions of dollars for the winner, and no expense was spared as each party laid claim to inventing virus-like particles.

Ian Frazer got on with his job back in Australia. He was kept up to date, but he had handed over ownership of any vaccine in the deal signed between UniQuest and CSL early on, and now Merck & Co. was their US partner, with so much to lose. Behind closed doors at its US headquarters, scientists were frantically using Ian Frazer's intellectual property to create a vaccine. It needed to be the victor in the patent hearing to open the door on the revenue stream that would flow once authorities approved it for mass use across the United States. CSL had unusually retained the obligation to prosecute the patent, which gave it enormous power in determining what to argue, when to argue, and how to argue its case. At Merck & Co., executives grew increasingly nervous. This was made worse when Merck & Co.'s main competitor, GlaxoSmithKline, signed up Georgetown University and Rochester University. Both GlaxoSmithKline and Merck & Co. had previously signed a non-exclusive agreement with the National Institutes of Health. So who was going to win? Merck & Co., which was relying on Ian Frazer and The University of Queensland? Or GlaxoSmithKline, which understandably wanted the other parties to come off with ownership of the HPV VLP?

In any legal battle, the points of contention eventually become obvious, and this hearing was no different. One point was whether you required the two proteins – late protein 1 (L1) and late protein 2 (L2) – to make the VLP. In Queensland's original patent, lodged in Australia, Jian and Ian and their co-authors talked about expressing both of these proteins. It stipulated that both proteins were required, a point reinforced by the pair when they delivered their crucial findings at the Seattle HPV conference in 1991. They originally did the experiment using just one of the proteins, L1, but had failed to see any VLPs. That's when Jian tried the L1–L2 combination. That slip-up – that they believed they needed both – was a stumbling block for John Cox and the team. (Both vaccines on the market today – Gardasil and Cervarix – are L1 alone vaccines.)

So much was riding on that original patent application lodged in Brisbane more than ten years earlier; it had been drawn up in a matter of days by Robin Kelly, in a bid to have it lodged before Jian and Ian revealed their invention at the Seattle HPV conference. Kelly used Jian and Ian's 'Virology' paper as the basis for the patent application; time hadn't allowed much else. Now, as the legal team was fighting for The University of Queensland's place in history, lawyers for the other parties were picking that paper apart. The patent had been filed on the basis of what they knew at the time: Jian and Ian had simply seen a VLP. The mechanics and the consequences of the finding did not become clear until later.

It wasn't the only stumbling block. Another revolved around something called the 'start codon' – a piece of information buried in a gene – for the L1 protein. Start codons tell the machinery of a cell where to start reading the gene information from, and stop codons dictate where to stop. Ian and Jian had started expressing the HPV16 L1 protein from its second start codon, and this was crucial for their invention. They had essentially found the starting point to express the HPV16 L1 protein. Until then, everyone had believed that the start codon for expressing the HPV16 L1 protein was in another specific position. The start codon was absolutely crucial to whether the Australian case would be accepted. Ian and Jian had worked it out on a scrap of paper, without really understanding its full significance, but now it was central to their claim, and the other parties were demanding more information.

Ian had found the two days of his testimony gruelling. The benefit of hindsight is a wonderful thing, and he made a mental note to document every step of his laboratory work from that point on. Emails had been unearthed and work books found, but some conversations had simply happened across a desk between Ian and Jian and he had to rack his brain to answer specific questions. The fact that Jian was no longer alive, (Jian tragically died in 1999, a few years into the patent hearing), made the process increasingly difficult. Some of his notes were in Mandarin and, while these could be translated, others were undated. If he'd been alive, issues could have been resolved quickly, but time had elapsed and records were incomplete. Opposing lawyers kept on about whether Jian had used a prototype HPV16 L1 protein, or a wild type, and questions were raised about the origin of Jian's samples; it was a secret that died with Jian, because no one actually knew where he had sourced them from. Where had he got the material from, Ian was asked. Could he rule out that it was prototype protein and not wild type protein that had been used? How could Ian, a scientist, categorically rule out using prototype, if it hadn't been tested and proved? Ian simply answered the question honestly, conceding that prototype might have been used.

As the hearing wore on and the lawyers battled it out, the scientists from all parties got on with their jobs, often talking and even collaborating. None of them saw this as a personal race into the history books. A VLP had been created, work was advancing on cervical cancer vaccines because of that discovery, and each year up to 275,000 women's lives could be saved.

Few scientists went into the laboratory seeking fame and fortune, but they all wanted to take science a step forward. So the legal wrangling was the domain of the lawyers being paid by their employers, and the fight over who would be first to market with a vaccine was a squabble for the big pharma. The problem was that neither GlaxoSmithKline nor Merck & Co. could deliver the vaccine without access to all the patented technology and that forced them to the table to nut out an agreement. It was a matter of more urgency for Merck & Co., because in August 2004 the United States Patent and Trademark Office brought down a preliminary finding against The University of Queensland and Ian Frazer.

While the hearing continued, and CSL continued to say it was confident of a win, Merck & Co. grew more and more nervous. It was due to launch its vaccine, called Gardasil, in a bit over twelve months, and had to settle with GlaxoSmithKline before that date, so it could access its patented technology. Merck & Co.'s money was running out the door as millions of dollars of investment became tens of millions and then hundreds of millions. The results for its 'phase three' clinical trials were due any day. GlaxoSmithKline was in much the same boat. So Merck & Co. went back to CSL, and the parties again ended up around the negotiating table. The University of Queensland was also becoming nervous that it could lose both the case and its promised pots of gold. After speaking with Ian, it made a call to accept a significant upfront payment from CSL in return for a reduced share of the United States market revenue when a vaccine eventuated. It was a gamble that paid off for CSL, which had backed itself. The university used the payment from CSL for the recruitment of more research staff.

On 3 February 2005, CSL announced a new arrangement that also included Merck & Co.'s competitor, GlaxoSmithKline. It was a cross-licence between the three pharmaceutical companies. The financial terms between CSL and Merck & Co. did not change, but – depending on the outcome of the patent hearing – CSL could receive royalties from Merck & Co. for an extended period, as well as receive separate payments from GlaxoSmithKline. The new arrangement meant that GlaxoSmithKline could access the intellectual property owned by The University of Queensland in return for making milestone and royalty payments to CSL. Whether or not The University of Queensland won the final interference hearing in the United States was now no longer as critical. The deal between all the companies had taken away the risk.

With that deal done, everyone got on with their job. Merck & Co., waiting for the results of its final clinical trials, put the finishing touches on its application to the US Food and Drug Administration for a mass rollout of vaccines. In Australia, where Ian Frazer had the patent sewn up, Australia Day committees were meeting in secret, ploughing through applications for the Australian of the Year. An application for Ian Hector Frazer was buried among piles of others, with the significance of his invention still the domain of the science world. And the science world was poised to hear the United States Patent and Trademark Office announce its decision on whether Ian Frazer, Jian Zhou, and The University of Queensland really did deserve the crucial patent. It made that announcement in September 2005.

Its decision was a blow to the Australian team. The Ian Frazer lab was not the first to make HPV VLPs and would not be awarded the patent, the Patent and Trademark Office ruled. It said the patent would go to Georgetown University and inventors Richard Schlegel and Bennett Jenson. Patent examiners had been won over by the other parties' claims that Jian had used prototype HPV16 L1 protein in his experiment rather than wild protein, the issue Ian had stumbled over when questioned. Their 1991 patent was therefore considered a 'non-enabling disclosure' – legal speak for being invalid, in this case because VLP technology based on prototype was not deemed usefully replicable. While they were able to retain their July 1992 filing date in the United States, they would lose their earlier filing date. Georgetown was awarded another filing date too – an earlier date of March 1992. This meant its date of invention was before The University of Queensland's. The winner had been declared. Queensland was runner-up, but there were no prizes for second place. Ian Frazer and Jian Zhou had lost: they were not considered the first to invent the HPV VLP.

Fifteen

The international argy-bargy being waged over the HPV VLP and any future vaccine didn't stop Ian from heading straight back to work. Science was about building tiny blocks, one at a time, that could be put together to make a difference, and from the moment the world knew about the VLP and began fighting over who invented it, Ian focused on the next building block – a therapeutic vaccine for women who had already developed cervical cancer. The VLP discovery, he knew, along with the work of other scientists, would lead to a vaccine that would stop the virus that caused cervical cancer. That wasn't a matter of conjecture. That would happen. But what about those women who already had the disease? A therapeutic vaccine, which could stimulate the body's immune response to attack cancer cells, went to the top of his must-do list. So for years – from when the VLP was first discovered in 1991 right through the US patent hearing which handed down its decision fourteen years later in 2005 – Ian and his staff toiled at that task.

He travelled to Madison in the United States in 1994 to work with oncologist Paul Lambert, who had set up complex mouse models, fought for grant funding to study immune system responses, and spent years looking at mice from every direction. The road to information was long and weary. It even took almost five years to reach one significant point: removing a skin graft from a mouse just by manipulating its immune system. It sounds simple, but that one step not only took years, but dozens of researchers, hundreds of meetings, and long weekends in the lab. The aim might have been a therapeutic vaccine for cervical cancer, but the steps along the way were painstaking and expensive.

As mice threw up new clues on how our immunological systems might work, Ian's research broadened out from cervical cancer to include skin cancers, but also head and neck cancers, genital warts, and herpes. He was interested in the possible link between different cancers. It was known that HPV caused cervical cancer, and the race to a vaccine was well and truly underway. But there was also significant data showing that HPV was involved in head and neck cancers, and some analysis suggesting it even had a role in skin cancer.

For his therapeutic vaccine for cervical cancer, Ian looked around his lab and realised he needed to recruit someone who had expertise in the culturing of skin cells. He picked up the phone to pharmacologist Nick Saunders at the National Institute of Environmental Health Sciences in the United States. Nick understood skin better than most, and the relationship between cervical cancer and some skin cancers was tight. The cells of the cervix where the cancers arise are the same sort of cells covering our skin, tongue and parts of our mouth: a particular type of surface cell.

Mice models were used to help determine how a therapeutic vaccine might work. For example, in the pursuit of a cervical cancer therapeutic vaccine, some mice were injected with tumour cells that were allowed to grow until a lump would become visible to researchers. They would then try and slow down or stop that tumour growth using a therapeutic vaccine. In other cases, the mice were therapeutically vaccinated before being injected with tumour cells to see if that meant that the cancer cells wouldn't get the chance to grow. The CSL-produced vaccine looked promising, and Ian Frazer and CSL embarked on a clinical trial to see if they could cure women with cervical pre-cancers.

The Brisbane women, all twenty-seven of them, had pre-cancerous lesions on their way to becoming cancer. That meant the trial, held in the late 1990s, had to be short, so that the lesions could be dealt with medically before becoming dangerous. At the end of the six-week period, researchers could see that the vaccine had created an immune response – which was good news – but it had had no effect on the lesions, which was bad news. There had been no difference in the tissue between those who had been vaccinated and those given a placebo. The outcome might have been a result of the short timeframe in which researchers could observe any changes, but, whether this was the case or not, it was back to the mice models.

While work played out like a long dance, with a step forward followed by a dip backwards, the children raced through school. Ian helped as much as he could but was away for weeks at a time, and Caroline certainly carried the burden at home. When the children settled into school, she ventured back into teaching, meeting new people, and striving for a work–life balance that was still very much influenced by her husband's heavy work schedule.

She met Linda Kleinig the day Jennifer started preschool. 'My name is Linda and my baby, Martin, died yesterday,' Linda told the group of mothers sitting around introducing themselves. Caroline and another woman took her for coffee, and it was the start of a friendship that both cemented Caroline's love for Brisbane and helped ease her husband's absences. Their children would have sleepovers, Caroline and Linda would shop together, and, each Friday after school, sausages on the barbecue at the local park would signal an early dinner. Linda helped Caroline belong, and she was intrigued by Ian. Her son James would come home after a night at the Frazers to tell her and her husband, Danny, that Ian wasn't happy because his rats had died. Other times he'd come home and say the rats were faring really well, and Ian was happy. Linda vaguely knew what Ian did for a living, but her son's ongoing stories prompted her to ask. The couples would get together often too, to play the murder-mystery game How to Host a Murder, where players take on the role of murder suspects. One night, as wine flowed, they tried to uncover the murderer in the episode Chicago Caper; Ian, dressed as a gangster, with a black hat, satin vest, and bow tie, enjoyed the wine as much as anyone. The nights would often end with no one really caring whether the right murderer had been identified.

In the lab, the therapeutic vaccine experiments continued and some things worked and others didn't. But one significant step in the right direction was noting the important role of inflammation in the body. It was becoming obvious, after years of research and as the millennium clicked over, that the area being targeted for an immune response against cancer cells needed to be inflamed, or nothing happened. That piece of knowledge alone was crucial, and helped the next discovery, when researchers used a skin graft model to understand why skin cells were so resistant to immune attack, and found that if you could knock out a particular cell type from the skin of the donor of the graft, grafts bearing tumour antigens would then come off – as long as inflammation was present. That step brought researchers closer to working out how the immune response worked. Then came the next little breakthrough, which told the story of how the cells did their job. None of it would make headlines, but with each step Ian Frazer knew they were getting closer to understanding the immune system, and that was a step closer to a therapeutic vaccine for those women who already had cervical cancer.

Over the years in Ian's lab, various immunotherapy tests bounced between mice and human clinical trials in a bid to lock down how the immune system worked. The cervical cancer trial was one attempt. Another was done, this time with genital warts, in China. Each experiment provided a lesson, not always a step forward. When staff would express frustration, Ian would tell them that each time they could rule something out, they were a step closer to a solution. The role that inflammation played in an immune response was crucial, because the degree of inflammation locally in the skin determined whether the immune system's killer T cells, necessary to eliminate cancer, could do their job or not.

The research into how the immune response functioned allowed Ian Frazer and his team to tell a story of how cancer cells proliferated, divided, and inhibited the ability of T cells to kill them. As work progressed over the years, the team found that at least nine separate steps were involved. Each had to be known inside out for the project to progress, and Ian understood that it would take years more to map out each of those steps in mice.

While Caroline and their three children were Ian's rock, his workplace provided a social environment he loved. He genuinely liked those he worked with, and was generous with his time and knowledge. They too liked their boss, who, despite a strong sense of self, carried no ego into meetings and never mentioned the international squabbling over the discovery made in his laboratory. Ian also tried to foster a work environment where people chatted freely and enjoyed each other's company. He didn't find socialising easy, but he realised it was important and his communal morning teas continued, even morphing into barbecues at his home. They were his work associates, as well as his friends. And that was particularly the case with Jian Zhou.

Jian and Ian worked together for three years after their discovery, before Jian accepted an appointment as assistant professor at the Loyola University Medical Centre in Chicago in 1994. That decision was driven by two factors: Jian wanted to branch out, and his boss supported that move; and funding for medical research in Queensland was drying up. The Loyola University offer was too good to pass up. There, he continued his lifelong goal to unravel the mysteries presented by HPV, keeping in touch with Ian and swapping information. Two years later he was back in Queensland, again working with his friend Ian, and now as the Lions principal research fellow and head of the papillomavirus virology unit at The University of Queensland's school of medicine. Ian welcomed Jian back with open arms. It was a partnership that would endure until the end.

And that end came far too early. A few years later, in late 1998, as Ian's children strode through high school and the patent hearing and vaccine trials dragged on in the United States, Jian became listless, easily fatigued, and his ankles kept doubling in size. Everything that had seemed easy now seemed hard. He felt like an old man in a young man's body. His wife, Xiao Yi Sun, worried about him, urging him to slow down and get more sleep. But he'd never learnt to do either; the tradition of those long nights in the laboratory in China had become his normal work schedule. Xiao Yi knew Jian had contracted hepatitis as a young man. It had been endemic where he grew up, but she knew that wasn't the problem now. Eventually Jian sought advice from Ian, who referred him to a specialist. But Jian was strong willed, and Ian was never quite sure whether his friend and colleague made any follow-up appointments. Then in March 1999, Jian travelled to China for work. He also planned to explore some homeopathic medicines, while he was there, in a bid to make himself better.

Five days after he arrived in China, Jian called his wife, complaining of fever and the flu. She could hear the tiredness in his voice. He just wanted to go to bed, he told her. Xiao Yi felt sick with worry. She wished she was with him. Their little boy, Andreas, reached for the phone, asking his dad to bring home a set of Lego. Each trip Jian would hide another surprise in his baggage for the little boy who made their world go round. This time Andreas was getting his order in early. It was the last conversation they would share. By morning, Jian's best friend, Roger Guo, had received a phone call from Jian's Chinese-based family in Hangzhou. He was dead, an acute infection stealing his future at the age of forty-two. The cause of death: septic shock.

It was a tragic loss. Andreas had lost his dad and refused to eat or speak for twenty-four hours before the funeral in China, only breaking his silence after he placed his favourite childhood toy, a fluffy tiger, in with his father's body before Jian was entombed. Xiao Yi's fairytale marriage had been cut short, her husband laid to rest in the same garden that they had sat in, as medical students, hoping they would grow old together. It was a marriage that stunned others, each doting on the other at work and at home. They would finish each other's sentences, sit for long hours talking about their work, and marvel at the life Australia had given them and their son. Xiao Yi believed she would never recover. Jian was also the family's main breadwinner, and his loss caused significant financial hardship. But perhaps the biggest tragedy was that Jian died before realising his own place in history. He knew that a vaccine would almost definitely follow his VLP discovery, but the hearing by the United States Patent and Trademark Office was still playing out and dozens of vaccine trials had yet to get underway. Every scientist knows an inkling is not proof, and Jian – who had spent his life working on something that would eventually save the lives of millions of young women – died unaware of the final influence of his work.

Ian, after talking to Jian's work colleagues in his Brisbane lab, arrived home to Caroline and their children with a heavy heart. Jian Zhou was his colleague but also his friend; a personal partnership that was built in another lab, in another country, at another time. They knew each other's families and worked together every day. And Ian knew they had been a winning combination. Two tall expats with a passion for science. Two researchers who had spent their lives looking at one little bit of science in a bid to make a gigantic difference. Jian eyed the specific, Ian the big picture. Jian's incredible bench skills gave Ian the vision ahead. Ian was devastated by Jian's death, but few saw him wear it on his sleeve. It wasn't his style; emotions were kept to yourself. Indeed, his eldest child only found out about Jian's death when Ian walked into the kitchen one morning wearing a suit, prompting questions.

Ian made himself a promise: if the vaccine came off, and it was still an 'if', the world would know the part played by his brilliant colleague and friend Dr Jian Zhou.

Brisbane's winter was biting, but Ian Frazer didn't care about that, or the onlookers staring at him as he idled the car engine at traffic lights. His son Andrew was in the front passenger seat and Callum was in the back, his arms wrapped around his chest in a bid to keep warm. Ian's latest fancy in opera was playing loudly, and, with the top of his blue Peugeot down, others were able to enjoy it too. Ian was driving his two youngest across town to school, and it happened like this each day. It didn't matter how far the temperature plunged, the roof stayed down. He'd always had a thing for cars, ever since he built the old A30 with his dad in the backyard of their Aberdeen home. The Peugeot was his current pride and joy and he believed it should be driven with the roof down, whatever the temperature. He could be swayed on the music though. Some mornings, he switched the opera off and turned up his latest passion in classical music. But today was definitely an opera day, and Callum wondered what the other drivers were thinking, knowing his father didn't given two hoots. That was just his dad, Ian Hector Frazer.

As Merck & Co. was using Ian and Jian's discovery to trial its vaccine, the three Frazer children continued to breeze through school and on to university without any pressure from their parents. Ian and Caroline believed they either did their homework or suffered the consequences when they arrived at class the next day. A love of science drove all three children, and Ian was quick to offer help. He loved it when Andrew built a pinhole camera out of a tea tin and some duct tape for a science project, and happily took him in to work to develop the photographs in a darkroom, explaining each step along the way. But while they didn't push their children, Ian and Caroline shared a view that each had to try their best, and on occasion were happy to resort to bribery to make that happen.

Jennifer had received a part scholarship in her first year of high school, on the condition that she achieve a minimum academic standard of eight A grades and two B grades across all ten subject areas. At the end of her first semester, she'd achieved nine As and one C for English, with the teacher noting that she was capable of doing much better. If she didn't improve that mark during the next semester, the scholarship would no longer apply. Ian sat down and negotiated terms with his twelve-year-old daughter. He explained how much money the scholarship saved the family each semester, and told Jennifer that if her marks improved he would give her an 'achievement bonus' of one-fourth the value of the saving. That amounted to hundreds of dollars, and, given the current pocket money rate was fifty cents per week, Jennifer needed no other motivation.

Caroline, with Ian often away, started working again. Finding a job hadn't been easy; like many women re-entering the workforce, her confidence was shaky after working at home for years. A friend took her by the hand to the teacher registration board and made her fill in the forms. Back in Scotland she'd taught maths and guidance for five years in a big comprehensive high school, and it didn't take long before she felt at home again in front of a classroom. At first it was supply teaching here and there, but it became more regular and that presented difficulties too. She had three children at school but wouldn't know whether she was required for work until they had left for the day. Sometimes she would race home, knowing that her three sensible children had let themselves in after school and were looking after each other, under the watchful gaze of neighbours.

Then, out of the blue, she was asked to apply for a job working with teachers to help students with behavioural problems. It was a steep learning curve, with her colleagues more skilled in the area of behaviour management. Caroline decided that she needed Australian qualifications, and set about studying a Masters of Education at The University of Queensland. She did it part-time over five years, while working. It made life at home busier, but also filled in some of the long nights when Ian was away. Eventually she won a permanent part-time position as a learning support teacher at Payne Road State School at The Gap in Brisbane. With legal fights continuing over the patent in the United States, Merck & Co. deep in vaccine development, and her husband frequently absent, she relished her work, remaining at Payne Road State School for almost a decade.

Money was still tight though, and Ian and Caroline budgeted carefully, saving for each family holiday and their children's tuition at Brisbane's top private schools. Caroline's return to education had been driven by her passion for teaching but also the need to boost the family's coffers. The children had to play their part too. On one occasion, when Jennifer wanted to join her high-school classmates at a space camp in the United States, Ian and Caroline insisted she get a job. She did, at a local fast-food outlet, and money quickly tallied up before, like most teenagers, she frittered it away. The deal had been that she would put up half the money required for the excursion, with her parents kicking in the remainder. But because Jennifer didn't keep her part of the deal, they didn't either – and she missed the trip.

Politics and current events flowed around the dinner table. Ian told each of his children that their vote was no one else's business. If one of them expressed a one-sided opinion, he and Caroline would sometimes make them take the other side of the argument, to balance up their view. Religion wasn't a big issue, but they were told that beliefs often differed and, even if they thought someone else's view didn't tally, they should respect it. Their parents treated them as young adults from the moment they entered the high school gates: their parental creed encouraged them to treat everyone with respect, to be polite even if they didn't believe it was warranted, and to treat everyone equally, irrespective of how different they might be.

That last lesson stuck in Jennifer's mind as she penned a note to her parents in her first year of university. She had struggled with her sexuality for years, and her parents knew that too. Now she was telling them, in a letter. It was an extraordinarily difficult letter to write, and she knew her parents wouldn't find it easy to read either. Jennifer knew her parents loved her and wouldn't shun her. They were open-minded, and put family above all else. But that didn't mean it was easy. She gave them the note and then went away for a few days, giving her parents time to digest it.

It was news that caused angst for Caroline especially, as it would many parents. Caroline loved her daughter and struggled with her decision, a move made harder when Jennifer moved interstate, began living as a man and changed her name. Ian struggled with it too, but his years of research in sexual health made it all much easier for him to accept. Eventually, he told his son that he shouldn't go around openly defining himself to other people. He should be who he was and let others work things out for themselves. It probably wasn't the advice anyone in the throes of liberation wanted to hear, but his son appreciated it, and the unity of their family went on unchanged, with Ian only ever referring to his three sons from that moment on.

It was a few years later, in the early 2000s, that Ian suffered a problem with his heart. It would race for no reason, and then beat normally; he couldn't pick where or when it would happen. It was diagnosed as supraventricular tachycardia – a non-life-threatening condition whereby a minor electrical disturbance in the element that regulates the heartbeat sets it racing. One of Ian's brothers suffered from the same condition. It provided a warning sign for Ian, and he reconsidered his health.

Jian had died too early, in 1999, and Ian knew how difficult it had been for his wife to find her way in the country that she and her son were now calling home. He'd helped her, standing up for her over superannuation and ensuring Jian's royalties from the VLP would be protected, but no one wished losing a spouse on anyone. Perhaps subconsciously, Ian's own health jumped up the priority list. One of his sons had nagged him about adding to pollution while driving to work. So to placate his son and improve his fitness, Ian started riding to work again; in the past he had often taken the shortcut, pushing his bike onto the ferry and riding it again at the other end. Not now. He decided to take up cycling with passion, riding where and when he could. Even the couple of close encounters with cars didn't dampen his enthusiasm, and his students grew used to seeing him walk through the doors of his office carrying his bike helmet.

Later, as he threw himself into work, overseeing projects in his Brisbane laboratory, keeping in touch with Merck & Co., and watching CSL deliberate over whether it would lodge an appeal to the 2005 US patent decision, Ian also challenged his three children, all of whom, without realising it at the time, were heading for careers in medicine. It wasn't that he didn't want them to follow his career path, but he wanted to ensure they had considered the alternatives. When Callum expressed an interest in studying engineering, Ian welcomed his son's decision. Callum is now a doctor. Andrew studied law as an undergraduate, despite the niggling in the back of his mind that he would prefer medicine. Now, like Callum, he is a doctor. His third son has also decided to study medicine.

Through their schooling, especially high school, they knew their father was a talented scientist, but they had no comprehension of what he had done with the creation, in his laboratory, of the world's first virus-like particle. Talk about his work didn't feature strongly at home during their teenage years, and, going to school in Brisbane each day, they were unaware of the millions and millions of dollars that had been spent in the legal battle to protect Ian's VLP patent in the United States. They had no idea that Merck & Co. was on the brink of launching a vaccine that would make their father famous, and rich. They had no idea, despite the string of awards he had started bringing home, that he had started a chain of events that in their lifetime could signal the end of cervical cancer. They didn't really understand what he was doing, or why he spent so many hours in his study at night and on weekends, and he never thought it was important for them to know. No one said anything at school, and Ian never expressed any frustration at the long, winding legal road. He just got on with his job. At home, he very rarely raised his voice. He laughed, but not as much as others. And even though he had lost his sister as a child, his best friend in Melbourne, and his colleague and friend Jian Zhou, no one can remember him ever shedding a tear.

Sixteen

Ian Frazer had shown little emotion when told of the verdict that he had lost the VLP patent in the United States. Fourteen years had passed since Jian Zhou had rushed into his office with a photograph of their VLP, and he would go to his grave believing they had won the race. Ian's lack of emotion reflected his inner feelings: it would have been better to win, but the patent spoils were over dollars, not people's lives. To him, it all seemed irrelevant now because a vaccine was being produced by two companies, the intellectual property spoils had been divided up, and Ian Frazer was well down the track of other challenges. In fact, he didn't even consider picking up the telephone in September 2005, when the result was announced, to suggest that CSL appeal the decision.

It was very different inside CSL's Melbourne headquarters. John Cox didn't take kindly to losing. His history with CSL dated back to 1962, when he was first employed as a cadet biochemist. Years later he was brought back by CSL's lawyer Peter Turvey to look after CSL's intellectual property, but Jian and Ian's breakthrough had taken over his life. He had worked night and day, travelling to the United States so often that at least two of the five years before the verdict had been spent away from home. And now the hearing was over. Ian Frazer had lost. So had John Cox. He didn't show it, but he didn't like it.

Unlike John, Peter Turvey showed his unhappiness. It was wrong. That's what he kept thinking, after being told of the decision. Despite the enormous pots of money that CSL had spent trying to take victory in the patent hearing, no one was laying blame at the legal team that prosecuted their argument, so this wasn't at the centre of his worries. The decision was wrong in spirit and, more importantly, in law, and shouldn't be able to stand. CSL should appeal, he thought, as he scoured the judgement for grounds.

CSL scientist Stirling Edwards, who had first found Ian Frazer and lured him into partnership with CSL, was furious, the decision irking him on a couple of fronts. During the early years, when the hearing was first collecting evidence from hundreds of witnesses, he had been working with Merck & Co., using Ian and Jian's discovery, to advance a vaccine. He had got to know Ian personally, and understood what made him tick. He knew Ian's lab deserved credit, and the crucial US patent. He also believed that Jian Zhou's family deserved to know that he had created the first VLP and now that legacy had also been stolen by this decision. But Stirling's frustration was driven by another factor too: he believed the United States Patent and Trademark Office had ignored a vital piece of evidence.

The University of Queensland's case had been knocked out because of the belief that Jian and Ian had used a prototype sequence, not wild type HPV16 L1 protein. But Ian Frazer had lodged their samples with the American Type Culture Collection early in 1992. Everyone knew that. It was mentioned in their US patent application, but John Cox had been advised by his lawyers not to test it. Ian, in evidence, couldn't rule out that prototype had been used because it hadn't been tested. With the round one loss, John decided to ignore the lawyers and source a sample to find out what had been used. Stirling Edwards and a team of scientists then repeated the experiment done in Ian's lab a decade earlier. To John Cox's surprise and delight, they found it was wild type protein, not prototype. This was crucial because it had been sourced from the American Type Culture Collection and its authenticity couldn't be disputed. The National Institutes of Health quickly sourced samples from the same place, but then had to report that John Cox's finding was correct. This sent the hearing into a spin, but the United States Patent and Trademark Office ruled it was inadmissible evidence because it should have been raised earlier. Stirling Edwards knew that they had evidence to refute the patent ruling. He realised the decision to appeal the finding would be made well up the ladder at CSL, but he went back to his work believing that CSL had a moral obligation to pursue the case. Ian Frazer and Jian Zhou deserved their place in history, and only an appeal could now give them that.

At CSL, views were understandably mixed. Millions of dollars had already been spent fighting the case, and the agreement the previous year to divide up the intellectual property spoils had provided an extra revenue boost for CSL. It was in a strong position, taking a cut of sales that would be generated by both Merck & Co.'s and GlaxoSmithKline's vaccines in the United States. It could just accept the judgement and get on with the next project, knowing its pockets would be lined for many years to come. But on the other hand, an extra pot of gold sat at the end of any eventual win because the seventeen–year royalty period would be restarted if the US Court of Appeals for the Federal Circuit found in Ian Frazer's favour and demanded the patent office reverse its decision. Lawyer Beth Burrous knew it wouldn't be an easy run. Over the years she had learnt not to second-guess what an adjudicating body might do, and she knew the US Court of Appeals for the Federal Circuit showed deference to a lower court, the fact-finding body. But she was primed to work on an appeal, if CSL decided for it.

The weeks rushed by, and then 2005 turned into 2006, with Ian Frazer being announced the Australian of the Year. Peter Turvey and John Cox burnt the midnight oil looking for further grounds for an appeal. They needed solid grounds, as well as an argument to convince CSL that further expenditure of millions of dollars, without any guaranteed outcome, would be worth it.

Their lawyers had told them that they could appeal on the grounds that the inventors of the Georgetown University patent had 'derived' the invention after attending the Seattle HPV conference in 1991, where Ian and Jian had outlined the VLP experiment. But they still faced a big problem: if they couldn't prove they had used wild type, not prototype, then they couldn't prove the Georgetown scientists had derived their invention. Georgetown would still be considered the first to invent using wild type. To John Cox, it was crucial that the appeal stress that Jian and Ian had used wild type. The lawyers disagreed. An appeal needed to address a *new* issue and that meant the debate over wild type would not be admissible. John, backed by Peter Turvey, was intransigent. And a compromise was reached. The basis of the appeal would be derivation, but the lawyers would carefully include the evidence that wild type had been used by the Australians.

Next stop was the office of CSL boss Brian McNamee, who was trying to build a global business in a company whose growth had been stunted by government ownership. McNamee was highly regarded by his team, with a reputation for listening. And that's what he did when Peter Turvey and John Cox bowled up with the argument to take the patent loss to a higher court in a bid to have it overturned. McNamee did the figures, knowing the revenue stream had already been carved up in the deal done early in 2005. The company was having similar issues in patent battles around the world, but the US market always stole the show. CSL was receiving royalties from Merck & Co., but a fortune more could be won if the ruling were overturned. If successful, the royalties would continue for a further twelve years. The figures lay on one side of a ledger; on the other was CSL's determination to back its intellectual property. Brian McNamee counselled John Cox that if you believe in your intellectual property you should support it to the hilt, and he supported an appeal. That appeal was lodged in September 2006, as Australian of the Year Ian Frazer's face dominated the debate about rolling out the vaccine to schoolgirls, and as Merck & Co. started rolling out its vaccine in the United States.

At 5 a.m. on 20 August 2007 – eleven months after the appeal was lodged and sixteen years after Robin Kelly lodged a patent application on behalf of Ian Frazer and Jian Zhou – John Cox reached across his bed and picked up the phone. 'We won!' It was a chorus of voices at the other end of the phone, sitting in a conference room in Washington. They had counted down the minutes to five, not wanting to wake him too early, but knowing he would want to know the outcome immediately. The judgement by the US Court of Appeals for the Federal Circuit was unequivocal. The court ruled that Ian Frazer and

Jian Zhou had disclosed a working example of their invention at the Seattle HPV conference in 1991. That was when the world learnt how to make a HPV VLP and The University of Queensland was entitled to the 'priority' date of July 1991 to claim the invention. This date came before any date allowed by any other party, so the patent was awarded to the Queensland inventors. 'We conclude that Frazer was entitled to the priority date of the Australian patent application,' the Court of Appeals for the Federal Circuit ruled. 'Since the Australian filing date antedates any date alleged by [Georgetown University inventor Richard] Schlegel, priority must be awarded to Frazer. We thus do not reach Frazer's assertion that Schlegel derived the subject matter of the count from Frazer's presentation at the Seattle Workshop, at which Schlegel was present.'

Beth Burrous was surprised; in her long experience she had not seen a superior court so categorically reverse a decision. John Cox, just as he had expressed little emotion at the first loss, smiled at the end of the phone; it had taken seven years of his life, and he liked to win. Peter Turvey knew that justice had been done; he felt as though he had won the lottery. It felt good to Ian Frazer too. By the end, he had read a pile of documents which measured five metres thick. He knew they had been first, and, while his Chinese colleague couldn't be there to celebrate with him, Jian Zhou would go down in history as part of the hardworking team whose invention allowed researchers across the world to hope that a vaccine for cervical cancer was within arm's reach.

By the time the court granted the patent to The University of Queensland, women around the world were being protected from the virus that causes cervical cancer. The vaccine had been rolled out in more than one hundred countries, including Australia, where schoolgirls lined up to receive three publicly funded doses in 2007. And it wasn't long before CSL began recouping, from its royalties, its entire VLP patent expenditure over the previous fifteen years. The patent win had created history for Ian Frazer and Jian Zhou and their employer, The University of Queensland, but it had also vindicated CSL's decision to continue to support Ian's intellectual property in the face of global opposition. The re-granting of the patent meant that CSL would receive royalties from Merck & Co. for seventeen years from the date of issue in 2009. In June 1995, the United States Patent and Trademark Office changed its rules to be consistent with the rest of the world: patents filed before June 1995 had a patent term of seventeen years from the date they were granted, while patents filed after that date had a patent term of twenty years from initial filing. Since Ian's patent was filed before 1995, and the patent did not finally issue until 2009, the patent will not expire in the United States until 2026.

CSL had invested a lot in research and development and winning VLP patents in Europe, Canada, Japan, and now the United States, but it had been a fantastic business decision. By the end of 2012, the vaccine globally had provided revenue to CSL of six hundred million dollars. A slice of that is then divided into thirds between The University of Queensland's commercial arm, UniQuest, and The University of Queensland's Diamantina Institute, and the final third is shared equally between Ian and the estate of Jian Zhou.

Ian Frazer would not be going to the bank, cap in hand, to ask for a second mortgage on his house ever again.

It took more than an hour in front of the mirror, but Ian Frazer was determined to turn himself into Gene Simmons, bass player for the hard rock band Kiss. It was the office Christmas party in 2005, and Caroline had already laid out on the bed her Cyndi Lauper costume. But Ian wouldn't be outdone. White make-up plastered his face, his eyes were coloured on, and his hair teased up, now pointed towards the ceiling. It was hot, dressed in leather, and the chains he wore signalled his location at any time. He stuck his tongue out. He liked hiding behind a disguise. Yes, Gene Simmons, with Cyndi Lauper by his side, it would be 'A Night To Remember'.

It wasn't the first time Ian would shock his staff by arriving at the office Christmas party in winning fancy dress. One Christmas he turned into the Arabian Knight, his hair hidden in a big turban, with Caroline dressed as a belly dancer by his side. He borrowed an earring from one of his sons and wondered about the protocol of having it in a particular ear. Another year he turned up as William Wallace in *Braveheart*, his face painted in a blue and white stripe, his front draped with a big wooden sword. It came in handy, late in the night, when he jokingly took on one of his Japanese students, who had come as a samurai.

But tonight, in a hotel in Brisbane city, Ian stole the show; in disguise, he didn't mind being the centre of attention, and that continued after the party when a taxi pulled up, looked at them, and then took off before they could open the door. Caroline looked across at her husband, a fifty-something Gene Simmons look-alike, who had enjoyed more than one drink, and then down at her own Cyndi Lauper outfit. She wondered whether they should start the long walk home, but Ian didn't flinch. The law required that a taxi take them if they were standing orderly at a rank, and that's what they were doing. 'The next taxi,' he said, 'will stop.' She admired his supreme confidence, even if she had to smile at how he looked. But he was proved right, with the next taxi stopping and whisking them home after the last party of the year.

At work, cancer remained Ian's focus. Its mysteries dominated the thinking in his lab, and, along with the discoveries being made around the world, a better picture was developing. Everyone was beginning to understand cancer better. Ian's mother was a three-time cancer survivor, having been diagnosed with unconnected bowel, thyroid, and uterine cancer. Indeed, cancer remains the most common cause of death in Australia; by the time we turn eighty years old one in two of us will have been diagnosed with it. But it was no longer the death sentence it used to be, and Ian wanted to help those statistics along.

It isn't that easy to develop cancer because a cell requires several mutations before it becomes a cancer cell; it needs a full hand of cards to turn bad, but three variables loom large in encouraging that. The first is environment, with sunlight, alcohol, smoking and radiation some of the most common examples of what can kick the process along. The second is simply bad luck, because every time your cells divide there is one chance in a million that any given gene in the cell will acquire a mutation because its copying mechanism is not perfect. But it is the third variable that continued to focus Ian's attention: a virus can also cause cancer.

It was widely believed that HPV played a role in cancers beyond the cervix – including about half of other anal–genital cancers, like penile, anal, and vulval cancer, as well as about thirty to fifty per cent of head and neck cancers, plus rarer ones, like the cancer you can get in the gap between your fingernail and your skin and in the corner of your eye. The complexity of it all meant that a single cure wasn't possible. Cancer is multiple diseases. Breast cancer might show as a lump in the breast, but it could be made up of one of five different cancer types, each created differently and each requiring different treatment.

Ian's immunology interest was tiny in the big picture of cancer research, and international conferences on immunology were flooded with others working on technology targeting tumours. It was a rich field of research, and his painstaking work continued to centre around vaccines to treat those who were already sick. The decade of research already completed, much of it with CSL, in a bid to find a therapeutic vaccine to treat women who already had cervical cancer, had given hope. It wouldn't be a vaccine that produced antibodies against HPV, as the cervical cancer vaccine did. That vaccine stopped the cancer-causing virus infection. A completely different way of thinking was required to treat a person who already had cancer: immunotherapy, which attacks cancer by changing the body's immune response to it. Here it is new 'killer' cells, not antibodies, that are crucial. A killer cell response was needed to destroy the cells already infected with a cancer-causing virus.

The cellular immune response in the human body is regulated, and that's important: if every time we contracted a virus infection our body made a pile of cells that were specific for that virus, eventually there would only be immune cells in our body, and no room for anything else. Regulation means the immune response is turned on and off so it doesn't cause damage. The challenge that immunotherapy throws up is that most of the time researchers are trying to do something with the immune system that the immune system should have already done by itself, and failed. This makes the task harder.

The knowledge gained over previous years was invaluable

to the next stage of research. Scientists had found that killer T cells went round and round in the blood, traversing all body tissues, but would only act if there were other danger signs in cells where they found an antigen. There had to be an alert signal they recognised, or they quickly moved on. Ian had learnt that some sorts of inflammation could provide that signal.

It was clear, therefore, that a therapeutic vaccine – one that could cure a cancer – would have to be very different from a vaccine that stopped the cancer from developing in the first place. Researchers needed to find the trifecta: inflammation, enough killer T cells, and a mechanism to overcome the immune system's desire to switch itself off. With the establishment of his company Coridon in 2000, this trifecta continued to focus Ian Frazer's attention.

Coridon, an unlisted company, was set up by Ian, Janet Caffin, who Ian had met through UniQuest, Jian's widow, Xiao Yi, and Jimmy Botella, a Brisbane academic, to own and milk a second discovery – codon modification – developed by Ian and Jian many years earlier. It is just as complex as it sounds, and both Jian and Ian believed this discovery would be at least as, if not more, significant as the VLP. In layman's terms, DNA is a code and the code words, or codons, tell cells how to make proteins. Several code words have the same meaning, but different cells are able to translate these codons more or less effectively to make the same proteins. So the codon that will give the best results in producing a particular protein depends on the cell the codon is working in. If you change the codon, you can improve protein production in the cells you want it produced in, and reduce it in others, allowing targeted effects. Jian and Ian came up with a method of identifying which codons did what in different cells, and took out a suite of patents over them.

At the same time, UniQuest was looking for an investment vehicle and did a deal, licensing those patents for a vast majority of equity in Coridon. Most of the shares were held by UniQuest, which also helped Coridon attract five million dollars, including money from the Liberman family in Melbourne. That money gave Ian's research a big kick along, to the point where they believed their codon modification technology could be used successfully in gene therapy to get rid of a very common non-melanoma skin cancer called squamous cell carcinoma. But at the starting gun, the race was called off when a child developed leukaemia after undergoing gene therapy in France. The three-year-old was being treated for potentially life-threatening 'bubble boy' disease at a Paris clinic. An investigation was immediately launched over whether the treatment triggered the leukaemia; both France and the United States immediately halted gene therapy trials, and that reverberated through medical and scientific communities across the world. With squamous cell carcinoma being successfully treated surgically, gene therapy was taken off Coridon's agenda. And with that one decision, the whole construct of what was behind Coridon had to be rethought.

While potential other uses for codon modification technology followed, it was a few years before enough funding flowed through the doors again to really make a difference. This time Ian Frazer turned his attention to using the codon modification technology for developing DNA vaccines, which, through the injection of engineered DNA, prompt a therapeutic immune response. The codon technology needed to be tested to prove it worked, but Ian's HPV–cervical cancer research remained covered under The University of Queensland's agreement with CSL and Merck & Co.: anything Ian's lab discovered would be owned by CSL, ruling out HPV for the DNA vaccine project. So instead they decided to focus on the herpes simplex virus type 2 (HSV2), with the knowledge that if a DNA vaccine worked for it, it would almost certainly work for HPV, and thereby cervical cancer, and perhaps other cancers as well.

While a therapeutic vaccine for cervical cancer remained Ian's goal, following on from his twenty years of research in the area, he thought the herpes path might deliver the answer faster. Herpes viruses are different from HPVs, but include two of the viruses recognised as being chronic infections that can cause cancer – herpes virus type 8 and Epstein–Barr virus. Chronic viral infections provide an ideal model for cancer: both are made up of cells that express non-self antigens that the human body should see but doesn't. So if a vaccine can be tested against herpes viruses, and the technology works, then it will also almost definitely work for HPV.

Several years of animal testing followed, with all the ups and downs Ian had learnt to live with. But in the end, the result brought a smile to his face. Their DNA vaccine was one hundred per cent effective in preventing a mouse from dying from herpes simplex, and eighty per cent effective in preventing a permanent herpes infection. In any terms, it was good news, but to a scientist with an eye on creating a human vaccine for herpes it was gold. The experiments were done over and over again and there was no doubt; indeed, the mouse was given a vaccine with five hundred times the lethal dose of the virus, and it survived.

That news opened the gates for the next step in the process: testing the vaccine in human trials to see if the response was mirrored. At the back of Ian's mind, he knew that mice can lie; they had lied to him time and time again. While they will show you things in the laboratory, teasing you with great results, the complete opposite can happen when the test is performed on people. For that reason, the cork has remained in the champagne bottle. If, in the future, the vaccine works in human trials, then Ian Frazer and his team know that it can probably be modified to work for HPV too.

While the cork remained in the bottle at work, they popped open in Ian and Caroline's new home after renovations were finally complete. They bought their new house in 2004 for the views of the Brisbane river, but it seemed like a big block more akin to an industrial warehouse than a family home, so they set about renovating it. This time, Ian left the hammer in the tool shed, and brought in architects. He had put a deck on their former home, laid down a concrete foundation and a floor, but, with money now coming in, this could be someone else's job.

Together, he and Caroline planned their new home and high on the list was making it eco-friendly. The toilets would flush with recycled water. Fluorescent lights would be banned and every light bulb would be LED. Enough solar generating capacity to meet their own electricity bills would be part of the plan. They even talked about separating from the main supply and running independently, but knew it was forbidden by law. A water heater would mean hot water was only generated when it was needed. A huge fifty-thousand-litre water storage tank would sit underneath the house. It was something they had never dreamt of – Caroline's relationship with it only strained after the devastating floods of 2011 sent the Brisbane River into their bottom level, and deposited wheelbarrows full of mud into the water storage tank.

Seventeen

By the time the appeal verdict had been handed down in 2007, awarding the HPV patent to the Queenslanders, the gold mine had started for Merck & Co., as country after country approved its vaccine and urged young women to take it up. But it had been a long, slow road, with the vaccine being tested on more than twenty-five thousand women and costing the company, according to insiders, hundreds and hundreds of millions of dollars before a cent was received in return. In Australia, both Ian Frazer and CSL's team were crediting Kathrin Jansen, who had become known as the 'German bulldog', for getting the vaccine to work inside Merck & Co.'s headquarters. Born in East Germany two years before the Berlin Wall was built, Kathrin had trained as a microbiologist and worked in Switzerland before joining Merck & Co. in 1992, about the time that the world was being told about the discovery of HPV VLPs in Ian Frazer's Queensland laboratory.

Kathrin had had an abnormal Pap smear in her twenties, but like many young women dismissed it, not really understanding what the consequences might be. Now, in her laboratory in Pennsylvania, she was all too aware of the havoc cervical cancer was wreaking across the world, as one of the top five causes of death among women. She didn't have daughters, but her bulldog instincts meant that creating the vaccine became a personal battle along the way, and she would not let go until she had won.

That moment had come years before the appeal verdict, back in 2001, when she waited with colleague Eliav Barr, who led the vaccine's clinical development, outside the door of a room where the results of one of the clinical trials were being discussed. The then president of Merck Research Laboratories, Edward Scolnick, was in that meeting but couldn't reveal all when he walked out. He simply smiled, telling Kathrin and Eliav to go ahead with further work and enjoy a glass of wine on the way home. That's when they knew their years of toil, sometimes late into the night and on the weekends, had paid off. The ups and downs of examining more than one hundred thousand specimens and assessing thousands of biopsies had been worth it. The nay-sayers had been put in their place.

Kathrin and Eliav, who grew up in the Middle East as the son of a cardiologist and an intensive care unit nurse, danced like no one was looking. They were still midway through the trial required to bring the vaccine to market, but this one would determine whether it went ahead or not. It had started three years earlier and was designed to look specifically at HPV16 because that was the most common and deadliest type found in cervical cancers. Alone, it caused about half of them. It was also the most difficult strain to clear. The trial's success, as they later learnt, was beyond their expectations: their vaccine was one hundred per cent effective. Ian Frazer had been tipped off about the result, but the next morning he turned on his television in a New York hotel room to hear it broadcast across the world.

The reason why this trial was so significant was not just its size, despite involving 2,400 women. It was significant because it provided the proof that if you immunise young women who have no evidence of HPV16 infections, and they are followed for several years, they will be protected from the virus and therefore the cancer that is caused by the virus. The virus, which could be spread through sexual contact, could not infect an immunised woman. The study was controversial, but if it succeeded it would be the ultimate proof that the vaccine would work. Kathrin was aware of that, and so was Ian. Alone in his hotel room, watching the news, Ian smiled. There were now no doubts.

It was 2002, a decade after Jian Zhou first raced into his office with his photograph of their VLP. At this stage the technology was still being attacked by other parties at the patent hearing, but a vaccine would get to market, and that offered hope to slash the mortality rate of cervical cancer, which continued to nudge 275,000 each year. But for Frazer, the announcement was also tinged with sadness. He picked up the phone and dialled Jian's widow back in Australia. While a vaccine would save so many lives, the scientist who had worked so hard to see this day would not. Xiao Yi Sun appreciated the call.

Kathrin started work on the vaccine soon after starting at Merck & Co. At the time, the plan was to produce the vaccine in insect cells, which teams in the United States and CSL in Australia were working on. Kathrin thought differently, going to her boss, Alan Shaw, and suggesting that yeast be used instead, in the same way it was used for a hepatitis B vaccine. Shaw backed the scientist he had employed, and Kathrin set about it, demonstrating that VLPs could be made in this way, and using experiments in animals to show how effective the VLPs would be as a vaccine. Merck & Co., with the international rights to manufacture the vaccine using Jian and Ian's VLP technology, ran the operation, but Ian Frazer's involvement remained crucial, and Kathrin loved talking to the Australian scientist who would answer any question she asked. He was the expert in HPV, and she learnt everything she could. It was complex and difficult, and with Merck & Co. writing an open cheque in a bid to be first, Kathrin was desperate they succeed. She'd dealt with many scientists previously, but Ian Frazer's open mind was welcome: he could have dismissed her as a novice on HPV, having never worked in that field. But he didn't. He respected her talents and wanted to pass on as much knowledge as he could.

With Merck & Co. now in charge, Ian moved on. His research turned to other cancers, and he had set up his own company to consider them. Bigger questions existed in immunology, and he wanted to answer some of them. His working relationship with Merck & Co. was terrific: he respected, more than most scientists, its role in trying to bring a vaccine to market. But despite Ian believing that the only way a vaccine would get to market was through a big company like Merck & Co. outlaying the funds, he was determined that one day it would all be done under one roof. The HPV vaccine was still being trialled, and he was building the next challenge: one day, he told people, the same facility would make the scientific breakthrough, test it on animals, conduct clinical trials, and refine it for patients. It was a hard sell, and he'd already started talking about a bench-to-bedside facility, but the cost was prohibitive; few politicians would sign a cheque for hundreds of millions of dollars. He plugged away telling everyone who would listen that it was needed: life-saving pharmaceuticals would come to market more quickly and not be subject only to commercial considerations. In the long term, it would be profitable too, because royalties would be kept in-house.

Developing the HPV vaccine took more than ten years, until 2005 when the final results of Merck & Co.'s clinical trials were made public. Ironically, that was the same year that the United States Patent and Trademark Office ruled against Ian as the VLP's inventor. All that Merck & Co. had been granted in its 1995 agreement with CSL was the rights to Ian and Jian's VLP technology and their patent. That didn't make a vaccine, nor was it a guarantee that a vaccine could even be produced. Merck & Co. carried a big risk load, having to show that the concept was biologically valid, how a vaccine would be produced, and how it could be manufactured on a mass scale. That research took more than a decade, and the challenges were magnified by the fact that Merck & Co. was determined to make its vaccine protect against four types of HPV: HPV16 and 18 caused seventy per cent of cervical cancers together, while HPV6 and 11 caused more than ninety per cent of all genital warts. Its aim was one vaccine that would act as an umbrella shield against all four. That meant Kathrin had to develop a cell-based expression system that could produce large amounts of high-quality VLPs for all those HPV types, presenting problems from the start because each type acted differently. And once one problem was solved, another surfaced. New ways to engineer genes had to be developed, and fail-proof diagnostic tests to measure infection levels needed to be built.

All up, more than thirty clinical trials would be held involving women all across the world, in a project that mixed medicine, molecular biology, and pathology. Even sourcing the women for trials was a finicky job. There needed to be geographic and ethnic diversity, and Merck & Co. used centres in Peru and Brazil, US colleges, universities in Australia, and women's hospitals in Asia to recruit a fair spread. Outside the science it gave rise to whole new industries too, with factories having to be built, and government health campaigns put in place to explain the novelty of this vaccine to the public. Firstly, three doses were needed for it to be effective, not one. Secondly, it would be given to teenagers, not toddlers, who were usually the target of vaccines. And thirdly, it was to be given to those who believed they were immortal and that cancer was something old people suffered.

Dozens of trials were held under three big phases, which ran from 1998 to 2005. The first phase focused on HPV11. Phase two centred around the proof-of-concept HPV16 trial, which showed it to be one hundred per cent effective. Phase three tried to simulate, as best it could, what would really happen when the vaccine was released, by trialling the quadrivalent vaccine, the vaccine that covered all four HPV types. This last phase involved girls as young as nine, and looked at the vaccine's effect on genital warts and cervical pre-cancers. Each of these phases involved several different trials, and each of the trials took years because participants had to be followed up over time. With the final proof in 2005 that it was effective, Merck & Co. bundled it all up and asked for government approval to release the vaccine.

It was in that same year that cross-licences were agreed on to allow GlaxoSmithKline to bring its vaccine to market using Ian Frazer's patent, and Merck & Co. to bring its vaccine to market by having access to the potential patents of other parties still sitting before the US patent hearing.

The following year, not long before CSL lodged its appeal against the finding that the VLP was not first created in Ian

Frazer's lab, the US Food and Drug Administration approved Gardasil in the United States and authorities recommended that vaccines be given to girls and women aged eleven to twenty-six. Nine- and ten-year-old girls would be vaccinated at their doctor's discretion.

Four weeks later, it had been approved in several other regions, including Canada, the European Union, New Zealand, Brazil, Peru, Taiwan, parts of Africa, and in Australia. Within six years – and still in its growth phase – annual Gardasil sales would reach over $1.2 billion.

Eighteen

Ian Frazer was momentarily overwhelmed. He'd just delivered the first cervical cancer vaccine in Sydney and was now jetting back to Brisbane to vaccinate Rochedale sisters Emma and Rachel McMillan, daughters of his colleagues Nigel and Denise. He looked out the window of the private jet to the expansive farmland fifteen thousand metres below. The plane had been chartered by CSL to resolve a clash: CSL had wanted the first vaccine to be given in Sydney, but the Queensland government was keen to ensure the world knew that Ian Frazer was from Queensland. So Ian administered the first vaccine in Sydney, to a patient close to that airport, and then was whisked to Brisbane by private jet. It was an experience he'd not had previously and, after escaping any security check and being told not to worry about turning his mobile off or keeping his seat belt on, he was now being offered a drink by the pilot, who had wandered back for a chat.

Administering the first cervical cancer vaccine was the pivotal moment in Ian's career. Until now, it had been theory. Sure, it had involved international scientific acclaim and a cupboard full of trophies. It was to make him a wealthy man, and he was now recognised when he ventured out with Caroline to do the shopping. But this day, when he first immunised two sisters against the virus that caused a cancer, was the moment he had worked towards his whole life. With the needle in his hand, he savoured the moment. His research had gone the whole circle: he had started out as the doctor wanting to save lives and had become the researcher who had, with Jian Zhou, helped create the technology behind a vaccine. Here now, he had it in his hand, ready to immunise the first child in his state. He sat back and thought about how each step had been harder than the first.

Conceiving the technology had taken years of trial-and-error experiments, but demonstrating it could work then became a bigger challenge, and securing the commercial interest required lengthy negotiations. Then the years of clinical trials. Now the vaccine was licensed, fifteen years after it all began, and he was a doctor again, about to vaccinate two young women, helping to ensure they would never develop cervical cancer. He felt an enormous sense of pride, but also relief. This vaccine would really make a difference, and not just to one or two girls. If adopted in those countries that so desperately needed it, the vaccine could make an enormous difference. This was the moment when he really celebrated the discovery made years earlier. Ian Hector Frazer, born on 6 January 1953, had done something really significant.

Seven months earlier, in January 2006, Ian Frazer had been announced Australian of the Year, and this changed his life more than the scientific discovery behind the award ever could. It also changed who he was, and how he was viewed by others. Overnight, he went from a private individual, happy in the largely anonymous world of science, to a public figure stopped by strangers in airport queues and shopping lines. Ian didn't find it an easy transition. At first he struggled with understanding why people would be interested in him, but the evidence that they were interested poured in: invitations filled his inbox, along with requests to speak at everything from business dinners to school awards nights. Within three weeks of the announcement that he was the 2006 Australian of the Year, his diary was jam-packed for twelve months. Grocery shopping became an event, and calls from the media would start before 5 a.m. He put enormous effort into ensuring that what he said was the message he wanted delivered.

The mainstream media would seek his view on the health issue of the day – everything from a new medical trial overseas, to funding for science and research. Science magazines lined up to request profiles of a man who had remained largely under their radar, despite the string of awards he had been gathering for years. Even cycling magazines wanted their piece of science's new poster child, who let it slip that he cycled to work each day. Ian felt owned by the public, but sometimes lost in the attention; after one three-hour plane journey, when his mobile telephone and email were turned off, he found eight hundred messages.

His family looked on bemused; and some of his sons' friends even hoped the association might help them in the girlfriend stakes. Being bestowed the award of Australian of the Year was a mighty one-day honour, he thought more than once, but the title also carried a heavy year-long workload. Ian tried to cheat the system once or twice, and get by unrecognised. He walked out of Brisbane Airport laughing to himself on one occasion, after a journey overseas. He had nominated, on his return immigration card, 'Australian of the Year' as his job description. No one had even noticed.

His surprise at the pace and public profile of the award was fed by the short time he had to think about what it would mean, before it was announced. He was given only a few weeks' notice that it might happen, but, from the moment he was told, he felt both compelled and proud to accept it. It had happened in an unexpected way too, with National Australia Day Council chair and former Olympian Lisa Curry calling him at home one December evening to let him know he was in with a chance. At the time, Ian was tucking into dinner with Caroline and a visiting US professor. A few minutes later Ian returned to the table, stony-faced but with his mind racing, and continued on with the dinner conversation, as though the phone call had never happened. That night, he tossed and turned.

Ian was working at the helm of the Diamantina Institute – a modern research facility combining scientific research and clinical trials – he had scheduled a trip to Washington, was about to go on holidays to Lizard Island, and had meetings set down in both the United Kingdom and the United States in the coming months. The conversation with Lisa Curry had been short, but now there were more questions than answers. What would it really involve if he were selected? How significantly would it take him away from his real work? It would be a wonderful way to sell science to the public, but was he best placed to do that? Did he want to live in the public limelight? The next morning, those questions remained. But nothing could now change the fact that Ian Hector Frazer, Scottish immigrant, might be voted Australian of the Year, and the prime minister would be making the announcement in January.

Of course the Scots have always punched above their weight

as public figures both in Australia and other countries. Andrew Fisher, who served as prime minister three times and started the Commonwealth Bank, hailed from Scotland, along with Prime Minister George Reid, and even the dominant Queensland premier in the 1930s, William Forgan Smith. Peter Dodds McCormick, the composer of the Australian national anthem, 'Advance Australia Fair', came from Scotland, and suffragette Catherine Spence was recognised on our five-dollar note.

In fact, our currency is a daily reminder of the roots of many of our past luminaries with strong Scottish heritage. John Flynn, who founded the Royal Flying Doctor Service appears on our twenty-dollar note, journalist Mary Gilmore as well as Andrew Barton Paterson, who composed 'Waltzing Matilda' feature on our ten-dollar note, with Nellie Melba, the legendary opera soprano, scoring the hundred-dollar note.

None of that entered Ian Frazer's mind ahead of the announcement, but he did consult two previous Australians of the Year – medicos Fiona Stanley and Fiona Wood. And he took their advice, booking a few short holidays for the year ahead, writing the announcement speech, and making a plan of how he would use his new profile, if selected. He jotted down three key goals in a notebook and promised himself to return to it as the year ended. Firstly, he wanted to win funding for his dream research institute where science could be harnessed from bench to bedside, and where reliance on big pharma would be reduced. This was a place to ensure that good science could travel all the way, as he would say, from bench to bedside. Ian's whole life had been driven by the quest for practical results: whether it was to dig a hole to a friend through the wall of his childhood backyard, build a car from parts, or create a vaccine. And the key to that in the world of research and drug development was to achieve the right relationship between the science and business communities, represented by big pharma – the half a dozen corporations that dominate the market for treatments and cures.

While Ian was a purist in the lab, he was practical when it came to the free market, starting from an understanding that pharmaceuticals can't be developed without the link between the scientist focused on minutiae and the drug companies focused on making millions, if not billions. There was no ideology in this, just pragmatics, with a fervent drive to get scientific research to work. He felt there was little value in lab success alone.

The reason the relationship had been important for Ian went to the issue of financial risk. The development of a drug or a vaccine could take years and cost a fortune – possibly without success. While universities were ideal hothouses for scientific thinking, they had never been the traditional custodians of such risk. So the partnership mattered. But Ian thought a Translational Research Institute would offer a better, more efficient, way of balancing that partnership, protecting the science from the commercial vulnerabilities of a corporation. It would be built in Brisbane, house hundreds of scientists, and develop and trial vaccines. It would also cost hundreds of millions of dollars.

Secondly, he wanted to promote science in the community by winning over the nation's youth. A long list of sports stars had featured as Australian of the Year previously. He didn't want to be considered a star in the same way, but he wanted young people to think science could be fun *and* a worthwhile option for study.

Thirdly, come hell or high water, he wanted to make sure his discovery was not just used in advanced countries where Pap smears were regular. Cervical cancer was the biggest killer of women in many developing countries. He wanted the vaccine to be taken up in countries like Vanuatu, where women could not access Pap smears, and it remained the leading cause of death. In the long term he wanted to see it adopted across Asia, Africa, and South America. But by year's end, he wanted it available in at least one developing country.

With a plan for 2006 now scrawled down in his notebook and a couple of weeks to spare before the prime minister would announce the new Australian of the Year, Ian, Caroline and a friend jumped on a plane to Lizard Island for a spot of snorkelling. Both Ian and Caroline would later think of it as the calm before the storm.

Cod Hole is a wonderful diving site on the northern tip of the Great Barrier Reef and home of the native potato cod. Ian and Caroline snorkelled, watching the huge cod below allow scuba divers to tickle them between the eyes. Some cod must have weighed almost one hundred kilograms. Caroline, particularly, was mesmerised; she'd never seen anything like it and wanted to touch them too. Ian made a mental note to give Caroline scuba diving lessons as a present, which turned out to also be a valuable present for him. After disappearing for a few days the following Easter for lessons – three months into his term as Australian of the Year – the couple had their diving certificates, and when the air became too thick with publicity Ian and Caroline would venture to the bottom of an ocean, where his mobile didn't work. He loved to get away, just to catch his breath, and that's what diving allowed him to do. It mirrored skiing and the solitude the snow offered. The passion for diving lasted beyond 2006, and, while Caroline eventually got to tickle the cod off Lizard Island and swim with sharks, the attraction faded when Ian's oxygen tank failed during one dive. He rose to the surface after buddy breathing, looking calm. He never doubted the emergency procedures he had practised down pat. But Caroline saw his face, understood the risks involved, and the next trip lacked the lure of the previous ones.

Back from Lizard Island, the announcement that the Scottish-born Queensland scientist would become Australian of the Year was made on 25 January 2006 in Canberra. Caroline sat in the audience, her children close by. She felt sick: proud that she had married this man who would soon be nationally acknowledged in a country they had both made their new home, but nervous he would not remember his speech. How would it be received, she wondered. Her hands were shaking as she took photographs in the late afternoon sun. None of them turned out.

I came to Australia twenty-five years ago because I saw it as a land of opportunity and a great place to pursue medical research, which is my hobby and my career, Ian told the audience. *My lifelong interest in vaccines has been guided by great Australian mentors, inspired by my students and assisted by my colleagues, friends and family. I particularly wish to acknowledge another great Australian the late Dr Jian Zhou, co-inventor of the cervical cancer vaccine. I believe that whatever we do in life, we should aim to do good for others. There's an amazing benefit from doing this: doing good for others makes you feel good too. I hope I can encourage you, in the singer Ben Lee's words, to 'catch my disease'. I look forward to meeting you during the year ahead.*

It was short, practised, and received well, and it wasn't surprising that Ian Frazer had borrowed from pop singer Ben Lee. Music had been part of him since the family sat around the gramophone in Aberdeen; he loved Led Zeppelin, Johann Sebastian Bach, and everything in between. It was the same with opera, a passion started by Mozart's *Magic Flute* and fed by the fun in Gaetano Donizetti's masterpieces, but Puccini's *Tosca* probably remained his favourite. He would make reference to music in his later speeches, but this one had to be short. He didn't mind that; he certainly didn't see the attraction in getting up on a stage and talking.

The next day – his first full day as Australian of the Year – the alarm was set for 4 a.m., and after a quick round of radio interviews Ian and Caroline were flown to Sydney. At the airport Ian pleaded with staff to allow his trophy on as hand luggage. The young counter assistant insisted it ran against policy and disappeared to seek advice, returning with a smile and a reprinted boarding pass made out to the 'Australian of the Year'. Ian smirked. This could be fun. It happened again on board, as the captain announced that the plane was carrying the new award winner, and his trophy. He was slightly embarrassed. Other travellers were acknowledging him for something that had happened fifteen years ago. He didn't quite know what to say, or even where to look, and was pleased that Caroline had come along with him. He was still the same person he had been a week ago, but it rapidly dawned on him that everyone in Australia would soon know about the cervical cancer vaccine. It would put pressure on the government to act on it, rolling it out to students across the country. He liked that. But the public adulation that came with the title made him feel uncomfortable. He wanted to sink into his seat.

On arrival in Sydney, he was told of his first public duty: later that day he would carry the Commonwealth Games torch into Sydney for the competition that would be held in Melbourne in two months. Hours later he climbed aboard the sloop *Kathleen Gillett* and took custody of the torch. Thousands had gathered along the harbour to see the magnificent fireworks promised later in the night, and, while Ian knew they were not there to see him, the sounds of welcome were deafening. He stood at the top of the sloop, the torch outstretched, and his mind wandered briefly. What would happen if he dropped the torch into the murky harbour below? He looked down at the water and held the torch more tightly. He'd been told that a message from the Queen was inside the torch, embedded into a chip. What would she think if the new Australian of the Year let that fall into the drink too? He was now gripping the torch as hard as he could. As the cheering grew louder and louder, he could feel the hairs on his neck stand on end. As people saluted from the shore, pride engulfed him. He had chosen to make his home in this country, which had now chosen him for this honour. Australia Day 2006 is a day that will always remain big in his mind. He smiled, alighting from the *Kathleen Gillett*. Back on land, it wasn't too long before reality hit him. It was a mighty honour, but it would also be a mighty job.

Until now, Ian had had little to do with the media, apart from the stuttering press conference he had given on AIDS many years before in Melbourne. He had learnt his lesson that day: always be in control. But it wasn't all that easy when everyone wanted a part of you. He was bemused by some of the coverage of his award too, including a headline in his wife's hometown newspaper back in Scotland, which celebrated the local woman's daughter's husband in Australia, and in his hometown of Aberdeen, where he was praised for saving mice from cervical cancer. But back here in Australia he found himself woken earlier and earlier each morning as the twenty-four-hour media cycle requested his views on everything from science to health policy. He did it because he thought it was necessary, but he didn't seek it. Because so little was known about Ian Frazer, most questions related to him and his beliefs.

But the vaccine got publicity along the way too, and he wanted that. And despite the positive coverage, he was prepared for someone to get stuck into him with the accusation that the Australian of the Year was promoting a vaccine that would make him rich. The year passed without that being raised as an issue, but he knew what his response would be if asked. He would receive funds through royalties, but the vaccine could also save up to 275,000 lives every year, and his lifetime of work had shown that money had never been a motivation in any of his decisions.

He was quickly ranked highly on most-trusted lists, ending 2006 as Australia's second most trusted person after medical colleague and burns specialist Fiona Wood on a *Reader's Digest* list. He was also on his way to winning every significant biomedical research award given out in that decade. It had started years earlier with the Australian Biotechnology Award, followed quickly by the Centenary Medal, the CSIRO Eureka Prize, and the John Curtin Medal. They were big gongs in the science world, but many outside that world had not heard of him until he became a regular on the news during 2006. While he would go on in following years to win more national awards, his first notable overseas prize was the William B. Coley Award he shared with Nobel prize winner Harald zur Hausen in 2006. To accept this award, he was flown with Caroline to New York to attend an upmarket reception in the Rainbow Room on the sixty-fifth floor of the GE Building in the Rockefeller Center. Usually the home of celebrities, Ian, Caroline, Ian's brother Neil, and Neil's wife Sharon had a ball, gobsmacked at the wealth that surrounded them. Afterwards, they snuck back to the bar in their own hotel, where Ian had a margarita, and then a second. Back home he had vowed not to have a drink before any speech, and even after delivering an address he was careful only ever to have one. Out of the country, just this time, he let his hair down.

It was while he was on this trip that he met Jacinta Stewart for the second time in his life. It was Monday 26 June, and he had promised to address a small group in the Monash Room of the Australian Consulate. He and Caroline set off to find the building on East 42nd Street, between Lexington and 3rd Avenues. Grand Central Station was just across the road. Ian talked to the group, mainly from business and university circles, and didn't at first notice the woman who had snuck in while he was speaking. But now she was on her feet, addressing him. She wasn't asking a question; she was making a statement, telling him how he had saved her life. He tried to recall an earlier meeting and asked her a few questions. She answered quickly. And then he remembered the skeletal young woman he had been asked to see at the Mater Hospital on Christmas Eve almost two decades earlier. It was in another country, at another time, but he had never forgotten the pain in her parents' eyes. They were desperate for help. And he remembered how he had diagnosed her with lupus. The past few years had revolved around accolades for the scientific discovery he had shared with Jian Zhou. But science was useless unless it could help people. He was a doctor, and he liked that Jacinta had reminded him of that.

By the time he returned from that trip, in mid-2006, Ian Frazer had his Australian audience in the palm of his hand. Politicians sought his opinion, the media gave prominence to his views, and the public now knew and respected him. But being a public figure was a talent he had to learn. He didn't like giving speeches, standing at lecterns, being the guest of honour, but it was central to the role of Australian of the Year, and he knew he had to master it. He only received coaching for that first speech: a senior journalist from Canberra told him the content was fine, but the delivery and length needed work. Ian sat down and wrote a shorter one, road tested it on the journalist as well as Caroline, and then learnt it off by heart. It was the first of two hundred speeches he would deliver that year, from Australia's red centre to the distant top end and the far reaches of Western Australia. He picked up quickly that most people were interested in science, but they lacked knowledge and wanted to understand more.

His confidence grew with each speech, and the response from audiences – ranging from Aboriginal communities to business groups, to public meetings where people told him their own cancer stories – was always enthusiastic. He learnt to add humour to entertain, as much as to inform, and at one point, while addressing a group of businessmen, he was shocked by how quickly he had learnt to slip into being a public figure when required. It was almost like donning a disguise, like dressing up for the office Christmas party. When he thought of it like that, it became easier. As the year went on, thick with speeches and public appearances, Ian also learnt other things: socialising became easier, vegetarian meals were less likely to put on weight, and the lectern could be used to convey the message he wanted to get out.

At school leadership ceremonies, he stressed that leadership was about changing how others thought, and that goals could be reached, despite any odds. He didn't pretend to be a great leader; he wanted to show by example what young people could create. But mostly he wanted to leave them with the message that they should never be constrained in what they think they can achieve: they should get out into the world and follow their passion. He told teenagers at graduation ceremonies across the country that his own story had been full of people doubting him: a virus can't cause cancer; a vaccine won't prevent cancer; no vaccine has been produced. Then, when he and Jian had proved them all wrong, the nay-sayers developed a different line of attack: it won't make money; it will cause promiscuity in the young; it will never reach the countries that need it most.

In each speech he tried to focus on the theme most relevant to the audience. He told people across Australia that a big chunk of chronic disease was directly attributable to our own lifestyle choices. He told one audience: *While twenty per cent of cancer can be attributed to infection, and therefore amenable to prevention through research, a rather larger fraction of all cancer reflects lifestyle – smoking, sun exposure, diet, and obesity – and should be prevented through behaviour modification at rather less expense.*

He called for more funding, better career structures for scientists, and more clinician scientists – and acknowledged the many doctors who chose to work in research despite poor salaries and the risk of not having their contracts renewed. Taking up the notes he had jotted down and kept privately since becoming Australian of the Year, he also pushed for better facilities for translational research, explaining that the discovery he and Jian Zhou had made fifteen years before had to be taken overseas to ensure it ended up coming back as a vaccine. *If we had been able to go the next step in Australia,* he said, *we would likely have increased the return to Australia from sales for the vaccine from seven per cent to thirty per cent, an estimated extra three hundred million per annum. We would have created more jobs in Australia. We might even have had the vaccine on the market sooner.*

A one-stop shop from the bench to the patient was needed. This sermon was for the benefit of the Howard government, ahead of its 2006 budget. He let them know it could improve its act, telling a Queensland audience that the government had done well in the past by increasing health research investment by twenty per cent each year for five years. Ian said the government was aware of the net economic benefit of investment in health – that there was a return of seven dollars for every one dollar invested: *So why, faced with this knowledge, is the federal government seemingly inactive at present?* he asked.

Politics had never featured strongly in Ian Frazer's life. A small-s socialist and a small-l liberal, he believed all politicians seemed pretty much the same; they got caught up in an unwieldy party process and voters' wishes were often ignored. But the year he was named top Australian there was no escaping politics. In Western Australia, Alan Carpenter replaced Premier Geoff Gallop, who quit, citing depression, Peter Beattie was re-elected as premier in Queensland, and Steve Bracks was re-elected in Victoria. The federal government's controversial WorkChoices industrial relations reforms came into effect, and mid-year the first revelations surfaced about John Howard having made a secret deal with Peter Costello in 1994 to hand over the leadership of the federal Liberal Party after having served two terms as prime minister. That was still being talked about publicly in December, when Kevin Rudd and Julia Gillard successfully challenged Kim Beazley and Jenny Macklin for leader and deputy leadership of the federal Labor Party.

But it was, ironically, federal Health Minister Tony Abbott who Ian Frazer respected the most by the end of his term as Australian of the Year. He'd battled Tony on a couple of fronts, and won on reason, he thought, but appreciated what he believed was the conservative minister's natural political instinct. He also envied the way Tony could speak in public, without notes and seemingly from the heart. It intrigued him, but certainly didn't lessen the struggles the pair would have before the close of 2006. The first one was over funding, with Ian determined to win money for his Translational Research Institute in the May budget that year. Peter Beattie was gearing up to put millions on the table, but it had to be matched by the federal government.

Ian also joined Tony on the annual Pollie Pedal – where politicians cycle between states to raise money for charity – in a bid to win him over. Ian arrived at the Brisbane start of the cycle with a black eye from a buster he'd received an hour earlier, and on the ride between Brisbane and Beaudesert, he put his case. A keen cyclist, he could keep up with Tony Abbott and told him why science needed extra funds. As they neared their stop, Tony gave him a promise of sorts, saying the government couldn't reduce medical research funding when it kept appointing medical researchers as Australians of the Year. But the wheels of government turn slowly and that budget, a couple of months later, didn't hold the pot of gold, despite some increases. It was the next one – in 2007 – that delivered one hundred million dollars for Ian's Translational Research Institute.

But while Ian had won over the health minister on funding, his support for the Gardasil vaccine did not come so easily. Mid-year, the Australian Therapeutic Goods Administration had approved Gardasil, but Tony Abbott publicly opposed CSL's proposed $465 three-dose shot, which would tally to more than six hundred million dollars over four years.

Tony Abbott joined a chorus of opposition, telling media he would not be 'rushing out to get his daughters vaccinated'. This angered women's groups, along with proponents of the vaccine, and fuelled a debate over whether he believed the vaccine might encourage promiscuity. The political climate on health issues was already emotionally charged with discussion over the abortion pill RU486, and Tony Abbott's decision to bring his own family into the vaccine debate empowered those fighting Gardasil. Arguments centred on whether girls would start to have sex earlier, the cost of the vaccine, and women's adherence to regular Pap smears.

Tony Abbott says now that his initial reluctance to publicly support the vaccine was driven by respect for the process: he wanted to allow the Pharmaceutical Benefits Advisory Committee (PBAC) to do its job without his interference. The PBAC had asked CSL to submit a cheaper proposal, and knocked back the application to make Gardasil free for all girls aged twelve to twenty-six.

Ian Frazer, the Australian of the Year, shook his head: the debate should be about saving women's lives, not politics.

He made an appointment to see Tony Abbott, and across the minister's desk, he explained why the vaccine had to go ahead. He told him that the vaccine had to be given to a girl before she became sexually active; that was why the age of twelve was appropriate. It wouldn't change the age she had sex, it would just provide protection against cervical cancer when she did. Cost effectiveness was not relevant because there were no alternatives, he told the health minister, and this vaccine could start saving lives now. Ian couldn't understand why a medical advance that had been applauded the world over – and which could eradicate cervical cancer – was so controversial. Ian doesn't remember Tony Abbott speaking while he put his case, and when he tells that story to friends now, he nominates Tony Abbott as one of the few examples he's seen of a politician who seemed genuinely willing to listen to expert opinion.

Of course it was Prime Minister John Howard who ultimately stepped in and delivered the go-ahead for the vaccine, announcing in November 2006 that Gardasil would be available for the National Immunisation Program the following year, from April 2007. It would be delivered to girls aged twelve and thirteen, but there would also be a catch-up program for those aged thirteen to eighteen. For women aged eighteen to twenty-six, the vaccine would be available for two years, through their local doctors. John Howard's intervention saw CSL come back with a lower price, and the rollout was locked in, a move the prime minister boasted would save many Australian women's lives, despite still costing $436 million over four years.

John Howard liked the tall Scotsman who he had announced as Australian of the Year at the beginning of 2006. He got talking to his parents at the ceremony, answering their questions about how they could eventually call Australia home too. Now he could see that the enormous influence their son wielded came from a mix of experience and common sense. People listened when he talked. Howard thought he was unassuming, and there was no doubting his intelligence. John Howard had seen Australians of the Year use their position in different ways; Ian Frazer was using it cleverly to sell science and win Australians over to his priorities.

On Gardasil, John Howard didn't need convincing, despite the price tag. A month earlier, his wife Janette had revealed for the first time that she had battled and beaten cervical cancer a decade before. That personal brush with the same cancer that Ian Frazer's vaccine could ward off was not the reason John Howard approved the vaccine, but there is little doubt it gave emotional weight to his commitment. He spoke from the heart when he addressed the controversy, and his reading of the political pulse was spot on: here was an Australian invention, receiving plaudits around the world, which could save up to 275,000 lives globally each year. It was a no-brainer, and his government would not be baulking at its introduction.

Ian ended the year believing that his title had helped deliver the national vaccine rollout. It also showed him the power of the media and how politics worked.

By the time Australia had committed to the vaccine, Ian was planning his next coup – and his focus was on Vanuatu. Across Asia, high mortality rates for cervical cancer were ravaging populations. No screening programs existed, and, by the time a woman was diagnosed, it was too late to cure. One in ten women could expect to die from the disease and yet many countries had not even heard of the cervical cancer vaccine. This played on Ian Frazer's mind; he felt that we needed to think of our neighbours too. It was also his final Australian of the Year goal: to introduce the vaccine to a developing country.

In the same month the government announced the vaccine rollout – November 2006 – Caroline's mother, Lorna, succumbed to a long illness and died, prompting Ian and Caroline to travel to Scotland, before returning a couple of weeks later as the shutters closed on 2006. Ian's last speech of the year was to graduating medical students at The University of Queensland; on his drive home, he mentally addressed the three goals he had set himself almost a year before to the day. Funding for the Translational Research Institute. It was in the pipeline, to be delivered in 2007. Tick. Improve the understanding and lure of science in the community. Tick. Vaccine availability in developing countries. He knew this might take a while, but the process was underway. Tick. He had the trifecta, and looked forward to 2007, when he hoped to sneak off the public stage and back into the laboratory.

Nineteen

Ian Frazer sat deep in thought. The last twelve months, as Australian of the Year, had taught him so much, and he was about to put it to the test. Now as president of Cancer Council Australia – a term that would run from 2007 until 2010 – he sat pondering the issue that sat on his desk. A private company had taken out patents over human genes and other biological material. The claims made by the patent holder, Myriad Genetics, included not only the isolated genetic mutations linked to breast and ovarian cancers, but to the proteins involved in the mutations and biological materials relevant to diagnostic tests. This would give Myriad Genetics monopoly control over the material. Ian didn't like the idea of someone 'owning' a gene.

Each person is made up of more than twenty thousand genes, and they provide vital information about us, including our susceptibility to disease. While patents had been issued over them before, there was growing concern about the practice. If a company was allowed to own a gene or other naturally occurring biological material, anyone else would be prohibited from using it for research, and Ian thought this could delay cures and treatments. Ian believed that the human genome was public property. He believed anyone should be able to patent a method of looking at genes, but there should be nothing patentable in the fact that genes existed – whether they were normal or not. The issue had come across his table courtesy of patent expert Luigi Palombi, who was trying to have the practice stopped. Unrest was also growing in the medical community about gene patenting. Ian Frazer decided it was a priority, and while the Cancer Council's many challenges would always be broad, he would lend his personal support to this issue.

Other issues that were naturally the domain of the Cancer Council – skin cancer, smoking, and bowel cancer – took up most of its discussions, and Ian Frazer went to countless meetings and breakfasts with politicians to argue the Cancer Council's position. These three issues were also the biggest focus for the Cancer Council's chief executive officer, Ian Olver. Olver, an oncologist, researcher, and bioethicist, knew Ian Frazer well. Their relationship was an easygoing one, built on mutual respect, an understanding of each other's roles, and a shared passion for the cancer council's objectives. Ian saw his role as supporting his CEO, and Olver welcomed the pragmatic approach the president brought to the table. Olver also knew he had Ian's strong support, and marvelled at how the former Australian of the Year was able to respond to every email Olver fired off within hours of receiving it – irrespective of what country Ian might be visiting, or what time of day or night it was. Others say the same; it was as though he never left the computer.

Skin cancer, which causes the death of 1,700 Australians every year, was always going to be a high priority, and Ian Olver didn't miss an opportunity to drive home the message that sun and sand carried serious danger. Ian Frazer, who had begun his own research into skin cancer, supported him. With one in four teens suffering sunburn on a typical summer weekend, the Cancer Council roped in cricket star Michael Clarke to front a campaign, lobbied government hard for funds, and even lined 1,700 towels along the beach at Bondi to show the stark reality of how many lives were lost each year to skin cancer. Each small win was celebrated – the take-up of 'No Hat, No Play' policies, programs to apply sunscreen to children in childcare centres, and to deck out playground facilities with shade. The solarium industry fizzled quickly, under the torch of media criticism, rapidly declining by thirty-two per cent over the three years to 2009.

To the public, smoking remained the Cancer Council's main focus. But with one in five Australians a daily smoker, and Australia boasting higher smoking rates than Sweden, the United States, Portugal, and Canada, it was harder to make headway. The Cancer Council knew that many smokers wanted to give up but struggled with the addiction, while young people, irrespective of warnings, continued to take it up. How do you destroy the myth that smoking makes young adults look more attractive, even more worldly? The Cancer Council joined other anti-tobacco organisations to lobby federal and state governments on two fronts: first, make cigarettes less obvious and attainable; second, make them less appealing, particularly to young people.

At the end of Ian Frazer's first year as president, the Tasmanian parliament passed some brave legislation: the display of tobacco products in all retailers except specialist tobacconists would be phased out over four years. Olver knew this would apply pressure elsewhere. At every opportunity the Cancer Council would repeat, like a broken record, that each year 7,700 Australians died from cancers caused by smoking. About the same number of smoking-related deaths came from other illnesses such as emphysema, heart disease, and stroke. The lobby was relentless, and community antagonism towards smokers helped to create a groundswell of support for change, with a key legislative victory announced by the federal government early in 2010: compulsory plain packaging for tobacco products. It would target the two issues central to the Cancer Council's fight against smoking, led by Ian Olver and backed by Ian Frazer: the availability and appeal of tobacco, particularly to young people.

But it was bowel cancer, and the chance to reduce its toll, that was top of the Cancer Council's agenda during Ian Frazer's reign as president. They wanted all Australians aged fifty and over to be screened for bowel cancer, which was stealing eighty lives each week. Ian joined Olver to lobby both sides of politics, reminding them that screening was also recommended by the National Health and Medical Research Council. It wasn't a cheap plan, the Cancer Council knew that, but screening prevented up to a third of bowel cancer deaths among the screened population. Extending it to all Australians over fifty just made good common sense. While some progress was made during Ian Frazer's presidency, the Cancer Council continued to lobby government to broaden its current screening processes. Eventually, in the 2012 budget, the federal government announced a timetable for delivering the whole program.

With forty thousand cancer deaths each year in Australia – and one-third of those preventable through lifestyle changes and early detection – smoking, bowel cancer, and skin cancer were always going to dominate the discussions during the time Ian Frazer was president. Indeed, those same three issues had been the focus when Ian had served as vice-president to Judith Roberts, and later when Hendy Cowan, who served as Ian's vice-president, took over.

Cancer Council staff liked Ian in the role of president. While he didn't see it as his job to interfere, he was a strong sounding board. Judith Roberts was struck by the way he made decisions; he considered the 'people' impact and his logic followed from there. He was always direct and could bring meetings back to focus when they started to meander. Hendy Cowan, a stickler for procedure, reminded his president a couple of times to adhere to the meeting rules, while Ian just wanted to get things done – by yesterday.

Cowan thought his president never really looked comfortable in a suit, and wondered how he had got to where he was with no semblance of an ego. Other Cancer Council staff thought the same. Ian would talk about his family if asked, and his university, even his research, but he didn't speak about himself. Some put it down to shyness, others thought he liked to be taciturn, but they were all aware of the influence he carried with the politicians who ran Canberra. They knew that senior politicians doing their research on a health issue would pick up the phone and call Ian Frazer, to ask his advice. And he was happy to provide it. He was also very keen not to be seen, in any way, to be using his position for himself. Hendy Cowan learnt that very early on, when he invited Ian into the swish Qantas Chairman's Lounge at Sydney airport. The two men had been in Sydney for a meeting and Ian was waiting to board a flight back to Brisbane. Ian looked uncomfortable, finally admitting that he was worried it would be construed as misusing his position. His embarrassment only grew when he ventured into the lounge to be recognised by everyone.

But while lobbying over skin and bowel cancer and the death tally from smoking took up the long days put in by Ian Olver, Ian Frazer's attention kept coming back to the issue of whether someone should own part of the human genome. Could he elevate the issue so that the public – those who had responded to him as Australian of the Year and had shown such a willingness to listen and learn – would want to fight it too? He wanted people to understand that gene patenting had the power to frustrate investigations into new cancer treatments, including vaccines. He needed them to understand that patenting a particular gene meant that researchers could not then carry out crucial work unless they had consulted the private companies that owned the patent their work might infringe. But he also knew, despite the efforts of a few politicians, including federal Labor MP Melissa Parke and federal Liberal Senator Bill Heffernan, that the issue didn't carry big political currency. It wasn't the talk of the day like interest rates, and, despite its importance, it was hard to sell as a crucial, urgent policy debate.

Ian Olver was in a mini-bus on his way to Canberra airport when biotechnology patent expert Luigi Palombi telephoned him. Luigi's passion came across quickly; he'd been interested in the issue for years, but his attention to gene patenting resurfaced when he read a report in the *Canberra Times* suggesting that testing for a particular type of breast cancer was under threat as a result of a patent being awarded. Luigi saw red and offered himself to the Cancer Council as an adviser on the issue. The offer was quickly taken up by both Ian Olver and Ian Frazer.

Ian shared Luigi's concern that women might not be able to be tested for a particular gene involved with breast and ovarian cancer because someone owned the test. The patents had been taken out by Myriad Genetics in the United States (the exclusive rights to the patents in Australia were held by Melbourne-based Genetic Technologies) and related to the human gene known as BRCA1, as well as BRCA2 genetic mutations. Mutations on the

BRCA1 gene were associated with increased risk of hereditary breast and ovarian cancer. While IP Australia, the national patents body, had been granting 'ownership' of specific human genes, the Myriad Genetics patent showed the real impact of the policy. *You can't block people from diagnostic tests because of intellectual property*, Ian thought. *How can a company treat part of an individual's make-up as its own exclusive property*, Luigi thought. They felt that no one had the right to claim they had invented genes or other biological materials that might be triggers for cancer. It was a powerful combination: Ian, a patent holder of something that might eliminate cervical cancer, Luigi, who held a degree in economics and a PhD in law, relating to the patenting of biological materials.

Together, they worked on raising the profile of gene patenting as a public health issue. Luigi understood the power Ian Frazer wielded. He wanted Ian to take a public position, to tell people about the consequences of commercial enterprise owning chunks of the human genome. Ian Frazer agreed, and in August 2009 he put pen to paper in an opinion piece that was published in the *Weekend Australian*.

As a scientist and patent holder, I can understand why clinical researchers seek to have their inventions patented, he wrote. *Individuals or corporations whose talent and hard work result in a useful invention ought to benefit from a system that protects their investment of time and effort – and their willingness to make the invention public – by ensuring their labour and creativity are rewarded.* According to Ian, patent law had been developed as *an incentive to ingenuity, to help make the benefits of invention widely available to further develop novel uses for the invention. However, patenting of a naturally occurring gene sequence and claiming the right to benefit from the use of that gene sequence by others fails on both counts.*

Its timing was perfect, published one week after a Senate committee began hearing on the issue. Right through the legal battle over Ian Frazer's patent, he did not stop communicating with scientists on the other sides. Science was about team work, with each team using what another team had discovered to advance its own research. That's how real advances were made, Ian thought, and that was the point that hit home in his first public support for a ban on gene patenting: *Science sits on the cusp of a surge in the use of genes in the diagnosis and treatment for major illnesses,* he wrote. *The collegiate tradition of sharing raw data among researchers must be allowed to continue unfettered so new technologies can be developed to benefit all.*

It wasn't just an issue in Australia, with Bill Clinton and Tony Blair announcing almost a decade earlier that gene patents should be banned. The thrust of their message was wider than genes, and enveloped the patenting of any natural phenomena that might impede scientific discovery. The case that had sparked attention in Australia had also been heard in the United States. There, Myriad Genetics was granted a patent, and this was mirrored by IP Australia. When a higher US court then overturned the patent, it was reinstated on appeal. In 2012 the US Supreme Court agreed to take the case for a second time. In Australia, the same fight has been unfolding before the courts, where Luigi has assisted Maurice Blackburn Lawyers, Cancer Voices Australia, and Brisbane woman Yvonne D'Arcy, who represents the human side of the debate. They challenged biotech companies Myriad Genetics and Melbourne-based Genetic Technologies, essentially asking the Federal Court to determine whether we own our genes once they are outside our body. The case focused on the patent over mutations to the BRAC1 gene. But while hundreds of gene patents have been handed out over the years, no Australian court had ever ruled on whether it was legal. For that reason, the Federal Court decision in February 2013 that allowed the private companies to hold a patent over BRCA1 was groundbreaking. The opponents immediately flagged an appeal.

Yvonne D'Arcy was first diagnosed with breast cancer in 1998, at the age of fifty-two. In 2009 she found she harboured a second and unrelated cancer in her breast. She doesn't fit the category of a genetic cancer sufferer – where the BRCA1 is involved – but she knows what it is like to receive that gut-wrenching news that you have cancer. For that reason, she says she is suing Myriad Genetics for those women without the power to fight, those women who might be carrying a gene patented by a company. At the moment, women can get tested for the abnormal gene, which often leads to cancer, but it remains a breach of the patents held by Myriad Genetics. While no other supplier of the test has been sued, it doesn't rule out the possibility, and Luigi wants that stopped, using both the courts and parliament to advance the cause.

But despite the rhetoric, the political will continued to only chug along for change. Luigi knew he had to build a political groundswell of support and knew Ian Frazer had the best chance to do that. Luigi, an articulate and educated advocate for the cause, admired Ian Frazer and his patient, even-minded, and unbiased approach. He also knew that Malcolm Turnbull had had a long chat to the cancer council president before standing up in parliament and arguing against the patenting of genes. He was one of only a few politicians demanding change, but he was a crucial and senior player in the mix. Yet Ian Frazer's support was a double-edged sword, which Luigi found difficult to reconcile. While his support to ban the ownership of genes was the springboard for debate on the issue in parliament, as well as on talkback radio, and as the promise of change grew, they had a difference of opinion. Ian Frazer didn't want to go as far as Luigi Polambi. It was a matter of degrees about what should and should not be legislated, about what could and could not be patented. But just as Ian Frazer's backing raised attention to the issue, his decision not to support the specific bill that ended up in federal parliament – the Patent Amendment (Human Genes and Biological Materials) Bill 2010 – hurt Luigi's argument for big reform, at least in the eyes of many politicians.

Both remain committed to changing the status quo in Australia, despite achieving some reforms in the Raising the Bar Bill 2011, an amendment to the *Patents Act 1990*. While tightening up some criteria, it did not address the central issue of whether a gene could be patented. Luigi will continue to bring cases through the courts and fire up our politicians to what he sees as gross injustice. And Ian Frazer remains committed to reform, continuing to attend meetings despite leaving the Cancer Council Australia presidency behind at the end of 2010.

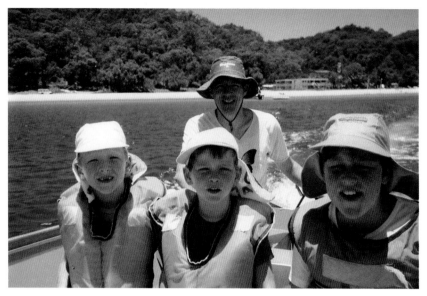

Ian at back with (from left) Andrew, Callum and Jennifer at Tangalooma near Brisbane during the Christmas holidays in January 1991.

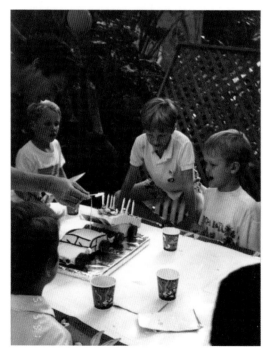

Ian with the 'garbage truck' cake he made for his son Andrew on his seventh birthday. The cake is one the many themed cakes that Ian has created over the years.

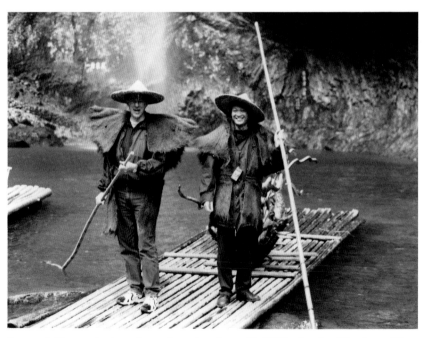

An image of a virus–like particle, called a VLP, which provided the basis for building the cervical cancer vaccine. This image is similar to what Jian and Ian witnessed, providing them with their major scientific breakthough.

Ian and Jian enjoying downtime in the mid–1990s in the Yandang Shan National Park in China.

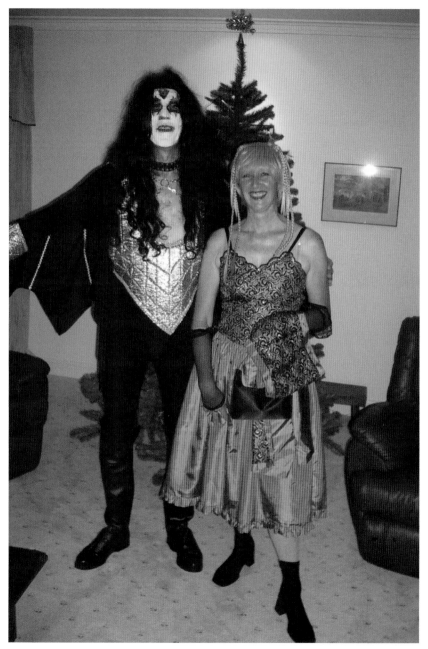

Dressed for the end-of-year work Christmas Party in 2005, Ian channels Gene Simmons, bass player for the rock band Kiss, with Caroline dressed as Cyndi Lauper, by his side.

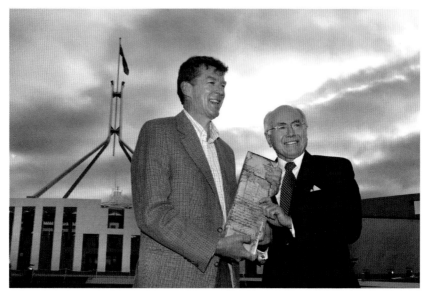

Ian with his Australian of the Year Award, presented to him by then Prime Minister John Howard, at Parliament House in Canberra on 25 January 2006. (University of Queensland's Diamantina Institute)

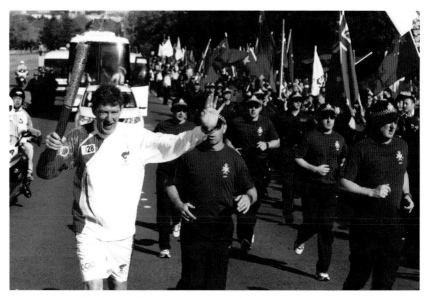

Ian Frazer in his leg of the 2008 Beijing Olympic torch relay in Canberra on 24 April 2008. (Photo by Renee Nowytarger/Newspix)

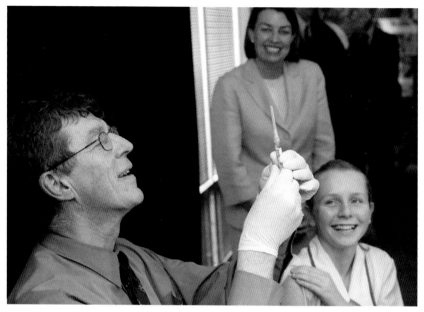

Ian preparing to give the first cervical cancer vaccination in his home city of Brisbane. Lining up to receive it is Emma McMillan. Former Queensland Premier Anna Bligh is in the background. (University of Queensland's Diamantina Institute)

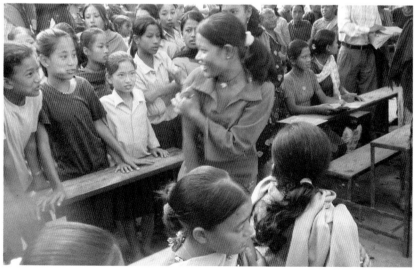

Hundreds of girls line up at local schools in Nepal to receive their cervical cancer vaccine during Ian's visit to the country with the Australian Cervical Cancer Foundation in October 2008.

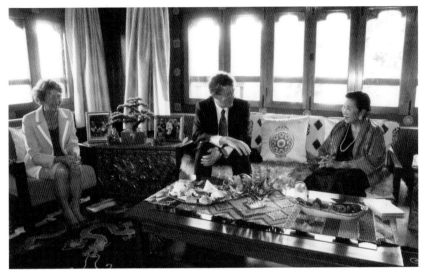

Caroline (left) and Ian meeting with the Her Majesty the Royal Grandmother of Bhutan at her palace in July 2012. By the end of that year 186,600 vaccines had been given to girls as part of a voluntary countrywide program.

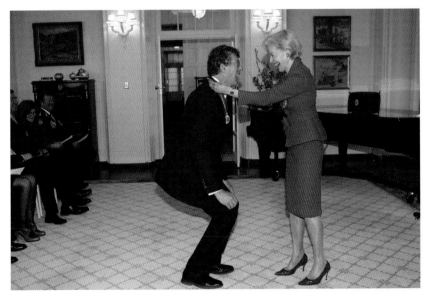

Ian receiving his Companion of the Order of Australia from Governer-General Quentin Bryce at Government House in Canberra, September 2012. The formality of the proceedings was noticeably lightened when Ian 'bowed' to accept the honour. (Kym Smith/Newspix)

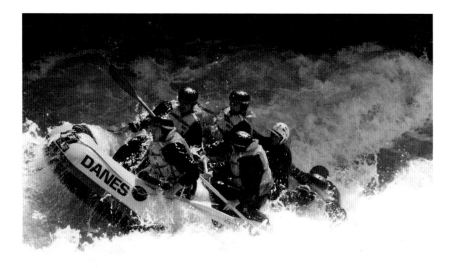

The Frazers enjoy white water rafting on Shotover River just outside Queenstown, New Zealand, 1995. (SmileCLICK Photography)

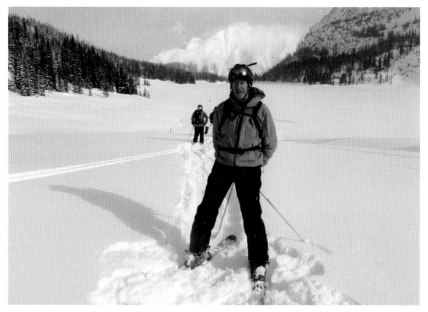

Ian waiting patiently to board the helicopter during a heli-skiing holiday in Canada in 2012. The seclusion of the slopes, as well as the adrenaline rush, provides Ian with some rare time out.

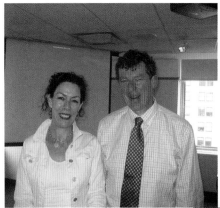

Former patient Jacinta Stewart with Ian in the Monash Room at the Australian Consulate in New York, 2006, where she finally had the opportunity of thanking the man who saved her life. (Jacinta Stewart)

Ian accepting an award from Lions International President Wayne Madden, commemorating his visit to the Diamantina Institute in November 2012. (University of Queensland's Diamantina Institute)

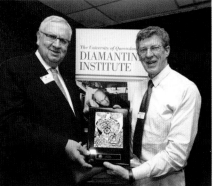

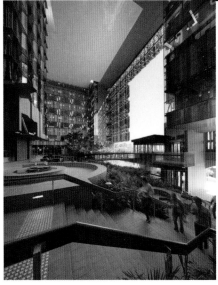

The $354 million Translational Research Institute in Brisbane opened its doors in 2013 with Ian Frazer as its Chief Executive Officer and Director of Research. With state-of-the-art research facilities the Institute will allow – for the first time in Australia – biopharmaceuticals and treatments to be discovered, produced, clinically tested and manufactured in one location. (TRI)

Twenty

Ian Frazer reached for his phone in the darkness. It was the middle of the night. On the other end was a representative from the International Balzan Prize Foundation, saying Ian had won their prestigious international award for his cervical cancer vaccine. In a fog of sleep Ian flipped open his laptop and did a quick search on the foundation to understand what he was being told. He had just won the preventative medicine category for 2008 and would be given one million dollars. He woke up quickly. There was only one rider attached to the winnings; half of it had to go towards funding a research project. A couple of months later, in November 2008, Ian and Caroline travelled to Italy to pick up the award, funded by the estate of the late Italian newsman Eugenio Balzan, part-owner of the newspaper *Corriere della Sera*, who died in the 1950s. Staying in luxury accommodation, being dined in private palaces and ferried around Rome, they had to pinch themselves. They had been to Italy before, the first time as cash-strapped university students, but never dreamt that Ian's work would one day turn their fortunes around so dramatically.

But money had always come a distant place-getter against the thrill of creating something new each morning. As Ian jumped on his bike and pedalled across The University of Queensland campus, over the Eleanor Schonell Bridge, and up to his office in the grounds of the Princess Alexandra Hospital, it was his next project occupying his mind. Now it was skin cancer, and the real possibility of creating a vaccine similar to the cervical cancer vaccine. With his pocket bulging, courtesy of his latest winnings, he knew the Balzan funds belonged to skin cancer research. His time with the Cancer Council was teaching him that Australians were not getting the message about the dangers of skin cancer. The number of skin cancer cases outnumbered all other types of cancers combined. Each year, almost five hundred thousand Australians were treated for one or more non-melanoma skin cancers, and the one that took Ian's fancy was squamous cell carcinoma. It wasn't as shocking as melanoma, but it killed a similar number of people. It usually struck later in life, where melanoma often cut down young people, but it could still creep, over time, into local lymph nodes and then into internal organs. It wasn't as quick or unpredictable as melanoma, but it was more common. And Ian Frazer believed it could be stopped.

People understood that radiation from the sun played a role in skin cancer, but Ian knew the immune system did too. The evidence was clear: the risk of developing squamous cell carcinoma increased more than one hundred times in patients who were chronically immunosuppressed. As a young medical registrar, Ian saw the cancer's toll on transplant patients in Scotland, a country not known for its sunshine. Then later, in Melbourne, he saw that his autoimmune liver disease patients also suffered squamous cell carcinomas. It was clear that a healthy immune system fought them off.

Years earlier it had been hypothesised that viruses could play a part in initiating some skin cancers, and a particular HPV had been isolated in a skin cancer lesion. But that hadn't shown causality. Finding conclusive proof lured Ian in. Technological and scientific advances meant that attempts to trace any connection had become easier. About two hundred different HPVs exist, and we carry many of them in our skin; one study even showed that a random piece of skin or even an eyebrow hair could harbour several different virus strains at the same time. Ian wanted to determine whether one of them might be responsible for the trip from healthy skin to cancer.

A few hints existed. In animals, papillomaviruses could cause cancers but were not found in the cancer itself. Scientists called this a hit-and-run mechanism, but did the same thing happen in humans? Another factor also stood out. The precursors to squamous cell carcinoma are sunspots called actinic keratoses. Most go away in time, but some persist and become cancer. When the immune system failed, the cancers were found. Were these sunspots caused by the HPV that triggered the whole process? The question went round and round in Ian's mind. The sunspots could be manifestations of an acute or chronic HPV infection that has woken up, and a healthy immune system kept them in check. Did a faulty immune system turn a sunspot into cancer? To answer the question, Ian's Balzan kitty would come in very handy.

Two obvious roads existed. The first was to take a guess at what virus was responsible, immunise against it, and wait decades to see what happens. This wasn't feasible, so the other option was to show that the area where the sunspots were found was associated with a particular type of HPV and then develop a therapeutic vaccine to trigger an immune response against that virus. Patients who were high risk – for example, transplant patients with depleted immunity – would then be given the vaccine to see if it protected them against developing squamous cell carcinomas.

Ian's working life has always revolved around the immune system, firstly as a young doctor in a renal unit in Scotland, and then later in Melbourne in his studies of HIV and genital warts. In Brisbane, his thirst for knowledge about cervical cancer focused on the immune system and how it worked. Each new project relied on the last; each big disease jigsaw was, in some way, tied to the next. Now, with skin cancer the focus, his team of researchers needed to understand how to rid the skin of problem cells. Slowly and persistently, they worked away inside Queensland's Diamantina Institute. Using experiments that Ian's lab had done previously, as well as new ones involving mice, they learnt that skin had natural defences that could switch off the killer T cells produced by administering a therapeutic vaccine. They found several ways to overcome this block and let the immune system do its job.

While a therapeutic vaccine was the end game, something else had to be proven beyond doubt before that step could be made. Clinical trials were needed to test whether an HPV infection on the skin increased the risk of developing squamous cell carcinoma. There had to be proof, not just educated supposition, along with evidence of how the human body's immune response also contributed to developing the skin cancer. Peter Soyer, inaugural professor of dermatology at The University of Queensland, would lead that investigation. Ian and Peter met in 2007, at a meeting of like-minded scientists set up by pharmacologist and skin cell specialist Nick Saunders, who had been recruited by Ian from the United States more than a decade earlier to help with cervical cancer research. As noted earlier, the cells of the cervix are the same sort of cells that cover our skin, our tongue, and parts of our mouth. Peter's interest was in skin, head, and neck cancers, and Ian's group was lacking an expert in those areas. Nick had worked with Ian since 1993, when his laboratory was based in the papillomavirus research unit, and he had moved with Ian as it grew into the Centre for Immunology and Cancer Research, and now the Diamantina Institute.

At their first meeting, Peter Soyer didn't see everything the tall, quiet Scotsman had to offer. He had nothing against him; Ian just didn't impress him immediately. But that changed quickly, and over the next few months they talked about the challenges presented by skin cancer, and the possibilities research offered. Not long after, they began working on a study to find proof that a virus infection on the skin contributed to skin cancer. Ian designed the study, but Peter ran it with funds provided by the Princess Alexandra Research Foundation. It involved two hundred squamous cell carcinoma patients in Brisbane aged between fifty and seventy years. The two remained closely in contact, and Peter saw Ian's total commitment to solving the skin cancer riddle. He admired Ian's work ethic too, even during meetings. Peter watched on regularly as Ian would send emails during a meeting, with one ear on the speaker; when the presentation ended, Ian would cut through with a relevant, difficult question, consider the answer, and then go back to his email. It was a lesson in multi-tasking at its best, Peter says, with more than a touch of admiration.

Science is slow. Mice can be used for decades to confirm one tiny fact. The cervical cancer vaccine started with the production of VLPs in 1991 and it was fifteen more years before it was on the market. The race to create a therapeutic skin cancer vaccine could take just as long. It's been broken up, with different researchers probing different pieces, not all of them supervised by Ian Frazer. The study into the presence of HPV in sunspots and the body's immune response is now being analysed. In another laboratory, under Ian Frazer's guidance, the results show that a therapeutic vaccine, at least for mice, is ready and willing. The next stop: human trials of a therapeutic vaccine to stop skin cancer.

Success would save the lives of thousands every year. It would also prove that the cervical cancer vaccine was not Ian Frazer's only lucky break: his theory that we can teach the body to fight particular cancer-causing viruses would have more far-reaching consequences. It wouldn't just be a vaccine for squamous cell carcinoma, but would offer scientists hope for flow-on potential across similar cancers on the surfaces of the body, as well as for bowel cancer, ovarian cancer and lung cancer. But, as always, the proof will be in the pudding, and Ian Frazer has learnt never to get ahead of himself.

Twenty-one

Dr Margaret McAdam didn't know Ian Frazer before 2006. She knew that the local Brisbane scientist had been awarded Australian of the Year, and while she was a busy general practitioner in the same city, their paths had never crossed. Apart from practising medicine, she spent as much time as she could out of Australia in Vanuatu, which she had fallen in love with after being introduced to it by friends. She loved the relaxed lifestyle and the locals so much that she holidayed there whenever she was able to, and made a whole new network of friends.

It was one of those friends, at a dinner party in Vanuatu, who took her aside and told her how cervical cancer was ravaging the island paradise. No screening programs existed, and by the time women were diagnosed it had spread through their bodies; the prognosis was almost always a death sentence. Margaret left the dinner party with an uneasy feeling. She admired Vanuatu women, their braveness, stoicism, and uncomplaining acceptance of life's circumstances. But she wanted to help them. She lived in a privileged position in a country where Pap smears were routine. Surely, if she researched the issue and sought the advice of medical colleagues, she could help. Home in Brisbane, she began looking into it.

The statistics were startling. Cervical cancer killed more than two hundred Australian women each year, which was much lower than so many other diseases, but its toll was much higher than the mortality rates suggested. Through screening more than 28,000 women were diagnosed with high-grade abnormalities; any one of them without treatment could go on to get cervical cancer. However, its real impact was in developing countries, like Vanuatu, and the figures there were staggering. More than eighty-five per cent of the 275,000 women who died across the world from cervical cancer every year were in developing countries. Screening in Australia had dropped the cervical cancer rate to one-tenth of that in Vanuatu. Ninety-one per cent of women in developing countries had never had a pap smear – and that's why so many died. By the time the patient fell ill, medicine was rendered next to useless. In these developing countries, it remained the leading cause of death for women. Margaret knew of the debate unfolding in Australia about whether to roll out an immunisation program to vaccinate every high-school girl, but it was the fate of women elsewhere that was weighing on her conscience. She wanted this vaccine to have a real impact in Vanuatu, where it could change a generation of lives.

The United States, like Australia and countries across Europe, had begun approving the vaccine, but that didn't help deliver it to those places most in need. Small pockets of rebellion were beginning to surface as US church, parent, and medical groups warned of the evils associated with it. The plan to mandate vaccinations for schoolgirls stole the right of parents to decide what was best for their daughters, they said, and promiscuity would rise too, as teenagers saw the vaccine as the green light to having sex without contracting HPV. Their objections would continue to rise, while deep-pocketed lobbying campaigns, including by Gardasil's maker, Merck & Co., tried to shut down opposition. Politicians can ignite the flame of discontent and that's exactly what later happened in the United States when Texan Governor Rick Perry added Gardasil to his state's required vaccination list. His decision was overturned, but not before headline after headline focused on the reasons why girls should not be given the vaccine. Perry, who stuck by his view that the vaccine should be mandatory for several years, reversed his position as he launched his Republican presidential bid, saying it was a mistake. It was an olive branch to the pro-family public policy groups that supported the vaccine itself, but not the compulsory nature of its distribution.

Much of that debate was still to unfold, and, back in Brisbane, Margaret McAdam was unaware of the brewing furore over the vaccine in some parts of the world. It certainly wasn't headlines in Australia, and she was concentrating on how she might stem the tide of cervical cancer deaths in Vanuatu. She spent a year researching cervical screening methods in poor countries. The World Health Organization was looking at a new technique whereby the cervix was viewed with vinegar staining and any lesions that turned white were frozen off with liquid nitrogen. Initial studies seemed promising enough. Margaret, who was not a gynaecologist, turned on her email and started trying to contact Vanuatu health authorities.

Those emails went unanswered. Vanuatu, despite being a premier holiday spot, shares all the problems of other developing countries. Communication is clunky, slow, and unreliable. Inexperience and less-than-ideal management can mire public health programs and send them into strife at any point. The logistics of running programs in Vanuatu can be overwhelmingly difficult. Money can run out halfway through the financial year. When fridges break down, there is no guarantee that medical supplies won't be dumped into buckets and rendered useless. Poor record keeping doesn't help either. None of this might be obvious on the surface of a country known for the happy disposition of its people. Despite widespread poverty and one-third of the population living on subsistence farming, its use by wealthy foreigners as a tax haven meant it would not qualify as a poor country for free cervical cancer vaccines. Those free vaccines, amounting to millions of doses, would be part of a special assistance program run by the big vaccine manufacturers for eligible governments and NGOs.

Margaret kept checking whether her emails had been answered. Eventually, she fronted the office of Vanuatu's director of health, Myriam Abel, ignoring the sign that warned that no walk-in appointments would be accepted. Something had to be done, she explained. Myriam Abel was all ears, and they determined they would work together. It was now a matter of deciding on a plan. Margaret consulted a group of girlfriends back in Brisbane, some medical colleagues. How could a cervical screening program and the HPV vaccine program that was now being rolled out free to schoolgirls in Australia be delivered to Vanuatu? One of her friends was blunt: go to Ian Frazer, the man who invented the vaccine.

A few hours later, Margaret tried to contact Ian. Her first attempt failed: same name, different person. So she tried again and eventually tracked down an email address and sent a plea for help to the right Ian Frazer, the serving Australian of the Year.

She did a double take when a response to her email popped up within a couple of hours. Surely he'd be too busy to respond so fast to someone he had never heard of. But Ian Frazer shared Margaret McAdam's view, and he knew that Vanuatu was the type of country where the cervical cancer vaccine could make a profound difference. Enabling the vaccine to be administered in a developing country was also one of his three goals as Australian of the Year. He was determined that something would be done by the time he handed over the reins to the next award recipient. Vanuatu also fitted his idea of the type of country that needed support: he knew it didn't qualify for a special assistance program, but unless help was given to the women there, cervical cancer would continue to rob the futures of so many women.

Ian agreed to help Margaret without even hesitating, and before long she was accompanying him to Canberra to talk to AusAID about helping, visiting the Wesley Research Institute on the way. She also called on Sullivan Nicolaides Pathology and other potential corporate donors. Six local gynaecologists volunteered their time too. It took months, of course, but Margaret found out quickly that Ian Frazer could open doors and empty pockets with a deftness she had never seen.

After an initial study aimed at looking at the prevalence of cervical cancer in Vanuatu, AusAID kicked in thirty million vatu (about $240,000) to help fund an ongoing cervical screening program.

Over the next year or two, Ian acted as Margaret's mentor, patiently answering dozens of questions, setting directions, reducing red tape and organising approvals. His involvement provided a robustness that Margaret knew any screening or vaccination program needed. A charity, Australians Helping Abroad, was set up to help with fundraising, research, and ongoing support to the Vanuatu Ministry of Health. Local medical staff were trained to read Pap smear results and identify abnormalities. Money was raised from a variety of different sources, including a duck race in Port Vila in Vanuatu, where people could sponsor a duck for five dollars. Cervical cancer vaccines were made by two manufacturers by this time – Merck & Co. as well as GlaxoSmithKline – and it was the latter that eventually provided, outside the big assistance programs, the vaccines to Vanuatu.

But just as opposition on moral grounds had sprung up in the Western world, obstacles also kept arising in Vanuatu. With more than eighty islands, it was difficult and expensive to convey the message to all women. Local woman Bernadette Aruhuri, who trained for six weeks in Australia to assess Pap smears under a microscope, returned to look for cervical abnormalities. She loved the work, knowing she was saving lives, but she also knew she had a big job on her hands. Women wanted to be screened: some lined up outside clinics from 2 a.m. Ten per cent of those tested were told they had abnormalities. Sometimes the unknown is easier to deal with than the known, and in many cases those women would refuse to come back for treatment, disappearing back to their villages to try bush medicine. But increasingly screening caught on, and a steady stream of women, mostly in their thirties, would front for examinations.

A pilot HPV vaccination program, which was run with Australians Helping Abroad and Ian Frazer in 2009, showed a mass vaccination program could work: 928 girls were vaccinated and ninety-three per cent came back for their second and third doses. This was a higher result than in Australia. There was no fear of vaccinations in these girls: no swooning, no fainting, just a desperate keenness to receive a vaccine they knew would help prevent them getting the disease that had stolen so many of their mothers and aunts and sisters. Each was given a coloured silicone wristband as a visible reminder to return for her later doses, and it had worked. The vaccine was administered by a district nurse through school and community groups in rural villages and in cities. Cervical screening was offered to their mothers as part of a separate program.

Ian Frazer acted as Bernadette Aruhuri's mentor too. It wasn't that he was going to put his own money into the program that surprised her. It was his generosity and patience in teaching her as much as he could. He was helping her save more lives.

With the support of the Vanuatu government, the HPV vaccination program is poised to take off on a national scale. With cervical cancer the second biggest public health priority after malaria control, the government has promised that all girls aged ten to thirteen will be immunised through routine school vaccinations. Australians Helping Abroad funded training in vaccine delivery for nurses, and awareness campaigns are underway. But each step brings challenges too, with some parents and schools still reluctant to allow the vaccine: some believe it will make their daughters promiscuous, not grasping that the vaccine must be given before the infection, not before the cancer, while others believe that HPV might be linked to HIV, and don't want anything to do with it.

Ian has put aside one million dollars to supply vaccines in Vanuatu; it's sitting in the Frazer Family Foundation. The Frazers are paying because of Vanuatu's exclusion from the manufacturer's special assistance program. Few people know that Ian and Caroline are funding these vaccines. But after upgrading their new home, buying a holiday apartment in Steamboat, Colorado, in the United States to indulge their passion for skiing, and giving each of their children a home, they have no use for the extra income flowing in.

Royalties from the vaccine go to others. In the case of Vanuatu, the one million dollars will supply the vaccine for five years.

But Vanuatu is one country, in one part of the world. What about other developing countries in the same situation? Nepal, for example. There were dozens of others, but each building started with a block. They had to pick a couple of countries and start the process of educating people about the vaccine. One night, Ian Frazer had an idea.

Graeme Lade, Australia's ambassador to Nepal, was used to people arriving at his office trying to sell him snake oil. They all had good intentions, but in two years he had heard dozens of different ideas, ranging from new orphanages to micro-hydropower projects, and none of them had eventuated. So when he received a call from a Mike Wille from Brisbane, who wanted to come and see him about a medical idea, he didn't hold high hopes. But, as always, he'd be polite.

Mike Wille, a well-regarded businessman, was a long-time friend of Ian Frazer, having sat with him on the board of the Princess Alexandra Research Foundation. Now Mike Wille was visiting Graeme Lade, explaining how he could help save the lives of thousands of local women with an invention that had won accolades around the world. Graeme listened and nodded, and appreciated his guest's enthusiasm; Mike Wille seemed in a different league from his other visitors. Mike's connection with Ian Frazer, who Graeme knew as the 2006 Australian of the Year, also helped persuade him. When Mike departed, Graeme checked up on what he had been told. He started his research with Google and within minutes was convinced that the idea might work. This just might be different, Graeme thought. This time the good intentions might turn out to be the miracle he'd just been promised.

The Nepal idea had surfaced a year earlier, in 2007, driven by Ian Frazer's ongoing concern that the HPV vaccine not only be available to the Western world. Nepal mirrored the mortality rates of Vanuatu and other developing countries: it was the number-one killer among women between the ages of thirty and sixty, and no screening programs existed. Over drinks, Ian and a group of friends had tried to work out how to get the vaccine to other developing countries. Waiting for countries to take it up was useless; many had never heard of it and those that had would never be able to afford it. Others had detected the little explosions of opposition to the vaccine in other countries and wanted nothing to do with it.

Mike Wille and his wife, Lenore, who was the former chief executive officer of the Princess Alexandra Research Foundation, and Linda Lavarch, former Queensland attorney-general, had known Ian for years, and shared his passion to have the vaccine adopted where it was most needed. Together they decided to set up a foundation, called the Australian Cervical Cancer Foundation (ACCF), with the sole objective of delivering the vaccine to women in developing countries. Mike's business contacts in Nepal led him to Dr Surendra Shrestha, a clever, well-connected local with a PhD in economics and a history of leadership in cancer groups. He was the ideal partner to help spread the word – and the vaccine – in Nepal.

Now won over, Ambassador Graeme Lade started making calls. So did Surendra. It was a messy process at first: Nepal's government was chaotic and not many people had heard of the vaccine, despite it being rolled out that year to schools in Australia, the United States, and countries across Europe. Graeme made more calls. Surendra kept trying to haul officials onboard, including those whose permission was needed to bring the vaccine into the country. While everyone expressed enthusiasm, no one wanted to adopt the plan as their own: the ACCF could embark on whatever plan they liked, implement it at the speed they wanted, but local help to deliver the vaccine, or to pay for it, was not the problem of the Nepalese health ministry.

Six months after the meeting between Mike and Graeme in March 2008, the vaccine was launched in Nepal at the Australian embassy. Four local girls – the daughters of senior medicos – received their first vaccine, with Graeme Lade looking on. A fifth girl chickened out at the eleventh hour. It was a humble start, with the four girls receiving their three doses over six months: the ACCF had a foot in the door.

Nepal's program grew as Surendra and his team continued to win over local hospitals and NGOs, and in October 2008, Ian and Caroline joined Mike and Lenore and others in a trip that vaccinated hundreds of girls through local schools. Ian's visit was crucial to securing another layer of support. He gave a public talk to an audience of government officials, medicos, and the media, as well as a separate talk to doctors at a teaching hospital. His appearances ensured that knowledge of cervical cancer and the vaccine was more widely understood 'and appreciated.

The following year – in 2009 – over three thousand girls lined up for the vaccine. In 2010 it grew to ten thousand, and then sixteen thousand in 2011 and 2012. The early doses had been donated in a deal involving CSL and Merck & Co. It was a generous move that fell outside its special assistance program for developing countries. The ACCF's costs – to open doors, run the program, and provide the staff – was financed totally through donations, chocolate drives, and chook raffles.

While earlier opposition to the vaccine across the Bible belt of the United States had centred around claims it would both increase teenage sex and take away parents' rights because it was being introduced as a mandatory vaccine, opposition now turned to its side effects. In the United States, despite the vaccine being tested in thousands of females and declared safe by the Food and Drug Administration, it was being blamed for everything from mental retardation to serious illness and death.

That campaign, fuelled by anti-vaccine groups, conservative bodies, and individual bloggers, bubbled along for several years until 2011, when Republican Party presidential nomination candidate Michele Bachmann criticised fellow candidate Rick Perry over his earlier directive to make the vaccine mandatory in Texas. 'I will tell you,' Bachmann told NBC's *Today*, 'that I had a mother last night come up to me here in Tampa, after the debate, and tell me that her little daughter took that vaccine, that injection, and she suffered from mental retardation thereafter.' While no reports of that case were ever received, it fired up opponents once again, creating headaches for those countries trying to roll out a national program. In Australia a lawsuit initially brewed after a Victorian woman claimed she suffered multiple sclerosis–like symptoms after receiving the vaccine. A Sydney law firm began to receive a steady number of inquiries, but no class action has followed.

The Royal Grandmother of Bhutan, Her Majesty Ashi Kesang Choden Wangchuck, would have heard of the hullabaloo happening elsewhere, but she was determined. The cervical cancer vaccine could save the lives of women across her kingdom. She handed her staff an old copy of the *Australian Women's Weekly* that contained a recipe for Anzac biscuits. She wanted them made for her visitors. Now the biscuits were laid on the table in front of her, and guests Mike and Lenore Wille from Australia, who had won over Graeme Lade in Nepal, were invited to have one.

Mike and Lenore had flown from Brisbane to Bangkok, and then from Bangkok to Bhutan after the Royal Grandmother, had organised their visas. Stepping off the plane, they felt like royalty: cars with flags, chauffeurs, and guards were there to greet them. And now they were sitting across from their host inside a palace, pinching themselves.

It was the same year that Bhutan, a country located at the eastern end of the Himalayas and bordered by India to the south, east and west, and China to the north, went from an absolute monarchy to a constitutional monarchy. The first general elections had been held, but no one could doubt the population's genuine affection for the royal family, or the influence it had. Happiness was important to locals, with even a gross national happiness index sitting alongside other considerations – like growth and public spending – when decisions were made.

Now, six months later, it was clear to Mike and Lenore what would make the Royal Grandmother happy. Women were being diagnosed with cervical cancer too late and were dying, she told them, as the Australians downed cups of tea and Anzac biscuits. How could she ensure that every young woman in the Kingdom of Bhutan could receive the cervical cancer vaccine?

Mike and Lenore were charmed; the Royal Grandmother's gentle voice and determination to protect those she felt responsible for shone through as she spoke. She wanted to be fair too; she didn't want some parts of Bhutan to receive the vaccine while others missed out. She wanted every girl to have the opportunity to receive the vaccine. Could they organise that? Please?

Mike felt like putty in her hands. 'Yes,' he heard himself say. 'Yes, of course we will.' He left the palace with a smile, but it wasn't long before the implications of what he had just promised became obvious. He had committed, he told ACCF chief executive officer Joe Tooma, to vaccinating every girl in Bhutan. Joe shook his head, but he loved a challenge too; firstly, he lodged an application with Axios, which ran special assistance programs to supply free vaccines from the manufacturers to eligible developing countries. In the process, he met Sean Lybrand, Merck & Co.'s regional director of vaccine policy. Sean knew where to go and who to talk to. Together, the pair returned to Bhutan to negotiate with health officials. The Royal Grandmother was championing the cause, and her will would win the day, but it was important for the government to be onside too.

Sean also thought that Bhutan stood out as the perfect developing country to launch a national vaccination program. It was small and contained, with a good record of implementing vaccination programs for measles and mumps, and it would be easy to track the results of the program. He took that proposal to Merck & Co. to argue that it become the first developing country in the world to vaccinate *all* young women for HPV.

It wasn't an easy process to navigate in either Bhutan, or Merck & Co.'s headquarters in the United States, where some executives had never heard of either Bhutan or the Australian Cervical Cancer Foundation. In Bhutan, negotiations were lost sometimes in translation. On one occasion it was over the extra five per cent of vaccines the government was demanding. It seemed a small addition, but would add tens of thousands of dollars to the bottom line; that money still had to be sourced from Merck & Co. Joe Tooma questioned officials again, finally receiving a clear explanation behind the request: the vaccines would be hauled up the steep mountains of Bhutan on the backs of donkeys, and every now and then one would slip and a load would undoubtedly fall hundreds of metres below. There was no way of rescuing the donkey, or the load, and that loss needed to be accommodated in the figures they were preparing.

With Sean's skills of persuasion, Merck & Co. supplied the millions and millions of dollars needed to vaccinate every girl in Bhutan aged twelve to eighteen for the first year. In close association with Ian, the ACCF agreed to fund the vaccines for the next four years. The Royal Grandmother continued to champion the cause, and was a driving factor in the 2009 pilot program, which saw 3,200 girls vaccinated, and the voluntary countrywide program the following year. By the end of 2012, a total of 186,600 vaccines had been given to local girls. Ian and Caroline have both visited Bhutan once, the Royal Grand-mother treating them like family.

With work in Nepal advanced, and the first national program in a developing country underway in Bhutan, the ACCF looked elsewhere, stopping at Kiribati, the island nation in the Pacific. With thirty-two atolls and one coral island spread over a massive 3.5 million square kilometres, distributing the vaccine to women across the islands was going to be a nightmare. This time the ACCF came up with the idea of motorised canoes that stash the vaccines in eskies, keeping them between the crucial two and eight degrees Celsius required during lengthy trips. The locals look out for their turn, with 8,400 vaccines – three doses given to 2,800 girls – disseminated so far. The ACCF's work is progressing in Vietnam too, headed up by the now retired former Australian ambassador in Nepal Graeme Lade. And East Timor – after an invitation from then president José Ramos

Horta – also remains a work in progress. So far the ACCF has delivered almost 260,000 doses of the vaccine since 2008. At an Australian retail cost, that would amount to thirty-four million dollars worth of vaccine. Joe Tooma's crew has done that with donations totalling $1.5 million.

The World Health Organization recommends that routine HPV vaccination be included in national programs where prevention of cervical cancer is a priority, where it can be given to girls before their sexual debut, and where funding is worked out. That's now happening, as countries like Rwanda implement a national rollout, with Peru and Uganda to follow. But China, the homeland of Jian Zhou, sits outside the requests for help. It is hell-bent on developing its own HPV vaccine, a process it began in 2006. Clinical trials are currently underway. It's not a reluctance to accept Western dictates. Pragmatically, if the Chinese can make the vaccine themselves, it will be much cheaper; and with a one billion–plus population, that is an important consideration. The other issue in China is the priority given to the prevention of cervical cancer. It is a serious problem, but not the number-one health problem, which remains the health consequences of smoking.

Nevertheless, the government wants a Chinese vaccine for Chinese people. Ian Frazer learnt that a couple of years ago when he answered his work telephone. The man on the other end was quite specific: the figure was five million dollars, and Ian Frazer would be required to teach Chinese scientists how to make their own cervical cancer vaccine. Ian Frazer wasn't interested in hearing much more. Money had never been a drawcard. He politely declined.

Twenty-two

The Hotel Vitale sits on the Embarcadero waterfront in the financial district of San Francisco. It's just across from the historic Ferry Building Marketplace. Designed by Heller Manus architects, it markets itself on being boutique and luxury. But the man who was about to walk through the front door could buy it in an instant, and Ian Frazer and University of Queensland vice-chancellor Paul Greenfield, who were standing in the lobby in March 2008, both knew it. Charles 'Chuck' Feeney, the Irish–American businessman who made his money on the back of duty-free shopping as plane travel began to boom, isn't interested in pocketing hotels. Known for his frugality, Chuck Feeney wants to leave his mark in a different way. Like Ian Frazer, he had put aside money for his family, and now wanted to use the rest to help others. Medical research rates highly on his philanthropic list, and so does Australia after befriending Australian tennis star Ken Fletcher decades ago. Ian Frazer and Paul Greenfield were now depending on both these interests. There had been talks along the way, but Paul Greenfield had the final plans tucked in a folder under his arm. They knew Chuck Feeney didn't dispense his donations willy-nilly. He had set up the Atlantic Philanthropies, a private foundation, in the early 1980s, and he knew from experience that you got more bang for your buck when your donations were matched by donations from governments or other institutions.

Around a table, the three of them sat. Chuck, wearing an open-necked shirt, slacks, and sneakers. Ian Frazer dressed the same. Only Paul Greenfield looked like they were there to ask for fifty million dollars. The clock ticked, as business seemed to be the farthest thing from Chuck's mind. He asked about their families, spoke about his wife, Helga, and wanted to know about the scientific and medical projects underway in Australia. Even US politics was on the agenda as the three men chatted for thirty minutes or so. That's how Chuck likes to do things. Nothing is frenetic. It wasn't casual, but certainly informal. Paul Greenfield, not knowing how much time Chuck Feeney had, steered the conversation to the point of the meeting.

A Queensland translational research institute had been on the cards for some time. A couple of options had been put up, but nothing had progressed. Chuck Feeney had promised money to the Mater Hospital, he had a solid association with Queensland University of Technology, and now he was being shown plans for a facility that would bind the institutions, or at least lead to a new level of cooperation between their sciences. He liked that. He was also very interested in Ian Frazer. The two had first met at Couran Cove Island Resort on South Stradbroke Island, when Chuck had owned it a few years earlier, and they'd enjoyed a beer at the bar. Then, too, Chuck wanted to know more about Ian and his ideas. Paul Greenfield watched their easy rapport as Chuck listened and Ian talked about the medical research and what it could mean.

Ten minutes later, it was over. 'Okay, I'll take a note of that,' was Chuck's only promise before leaving. But Ian and Paul both thought the same thing: nothing was signed, sealed and delivered, they didn't yet have the matching funds, but Chuck had sounded very interested and had taken the documents.

Months passed, along with due diligence, further meetings between the Atlantic Philanthropies and those working out the finances, and further appeals for donations, but the commitment finally came. It was an enormous relief. With Chuck, Ian and Paul knew, you could never be sure. But it had happened: Chuck Feeney was good for fifty million dollars. Paul Greenfield knew that Ian and his passion for progressing science had been the winning factor.

Paul Greenfield had met Ian years earlier, when the VLP was first being commercialised. He was struck then by Ian's balance: he could be a researcher and research leader at the same time. He was actively involved in determining how the VLP was commercialised, and the deal remains the biggest commercialisation ever done by the university. In fact, the VLP led to increased interest from overseas companies in Australian biotechnology. But Ian also had an ability to step back, even from his own arguments, to provide a critical view. Whether it was a faculty issue or an issue relating to research, he could paint an overall picture without being partisan. In meetings, Paul noticed that Ian never dominated. He listened. He contributed. He would always give his view, and he liked people to challenge his opinion too. But he wanted each meeting to deliver something; that was clear. It was also clear when frustrations kept hampering the plan to build Queensland's Translational Research Institute. Matching donations meant that the state and federal governments needed to dig deep, and that was a hard sell. Ian chipped away with the same focus he had shown as Australian of the Year.

Building and growing things are the two tasks that Ian loves more than anything. The lemon tree that he and Caroline had bought for their balcony became the source of his signature dish, lemon meringue pie. It started out as a little potted plant, had been nourished and fed, and now had outgrown its pot three times. Twice a year it would reward them with a crop of between twenty and thirty lemons. It looked nice, but for Ian it had to have a function too. So he baked the lemons into pies. (You can try Ian's lemon meringue pie; the recipe is on page 236.)

Just as he would spend hours building anything as a child, the ability and desire to build became the driving force behind his success as a scientist. Running university skiing holidays developed into organising international HPV conferences. The sponsorship he got for The University of Edinburgh medical year book became tens of millions of dollars in donations off the likes of Chuck Feeney. The HPV VLP discovery grew into a vaccine that can end cervical cancer across the world. And the tiny room that he moved into in 1985 in the basement of the Princess Alexandra Hospital, jokingly referred to by Ian and his few staff as a broom cupboard, would in 2012 become the Translational Research Institute (TRI), a 32,000-square-metre facility and one of the only buildings of its kind in the world. In an agreement between The University of Queensland, Queensland University of Technology, Mater Medical Research Institute, Princess Alexandra Hospital and the Queensland government, the TRI will be a one-stop science shop, where discoveries can be made, tested and manufactured in-house.

Ian Frazer sits at the top, as chief executive officer and research director.

Appointing Ian to that post wasn't a hard choice for TRI chairman David Watson. David knew the chance of finding someone of Ian's calibre who could overcome Ian's advantage – of working on the project, fighting for funds and understanding the background – was extremely unlikely. Watson's board agreed, and in July 2011 Ian was given the chief executive officer position. The building wouldn't open for more than a year.

The appointment was no surprise to Ian. He had worked on creating a building of this type for years, jotting down in notebooks how it could work and who might give money. The impetus for that was the cervical cancer vaccine. He knew he had to hand it over to commercial enterprise to develop; a university was not funded well enough to take a punt on something that might not work. But he also knew, if he had kept the technology in-house, that the vaccine would have been a cash cow for the university, and future research, for decades. It was a commercial awakening for the university and its commercial arm, UniQuest, and while more would now be done to take new technology further before handing it over, Ian and the university had little choice back in the early 1990s. A bench-to-bedside facility had long been Ian's aim; it was always just a matter of trying to make it happen.

When Ian first arrived in Brisbane, he used the tiny room he had been given as the motivation to ask for more funding. The few staff based there had to squeeze past each other, and it wasn't long before Ian was asking for funds from the Lions Kidney and Medical Research Foundation. It agreed, allowing him to have an extra scientist, and he determined he would never forget that. Indeed, it signalled the beginning of his ongoing interest in the Lions Club. But within a couple of years, as good academic papers coming out of his lab attracted recognition, he needed bigger premises, and it wasn't long before he upgraded to the Centre for Immunology and Cancer Research.

All along, while ensuring the buildings grew bigger, he made sure the science matched them. He'd lured Bob Tindle, the expert in monoclonal antibodies, out from the United Kingdom in 1987 to join him in a position funded by the Lions Kidney and Medical Research Foundation. Then Ranjeny Thomas, who returned to Australia from the United States as a senior lecturer in rheumatology, joined Ian's Centre for Immunology and Cancer Research as deputy director. In 2000 the new Princess Alexandra Hospital opened, and his centre moved to a larger wing in the hospital.

Ian was already thinking of the next move and the new programs he could launch. He added scientists like Matt Brown, who he convinced to come back from Oxford and who took on the post of professor of immunogenetics for Ian. The recruitments were helped by the money that began to pour into the university courtesy of the first big payment from Merck & Co. for the cervical cancer vaccine. Another hiring took more work, but Ian was eventually able to convince talented Oxford biomedical engineer Mark Kendall to return to Brisbane as a thirty-three-year-old professor.

In 2008 Ian's centre was renamed the University of Queensland Diamantina Institute when it became an independent faculty-level institute. A plan went forward to call it the Frazer Institute, but this was hit on the head by Ian immediately. Buildings were named after dead people, he told friends, and he was a long way short of that. Ranjeny Thomas became the Diamantina Institute's deputy, under Ian Frazer. The Translational Research Institute was already on the drawing board too, and, despite running the Diamantina Institute, Ian was focused on getting the new building, and more cooperation between different laboratories, up and running as soon as possible.

Money moved things, and Ian had used every opportunity since being appointed Australian of the Year to request help for his translational research facility. On his bike ride with Tony Abbott that year, he asked the health minister for $100 million. Eventually the Australian government handed over $140 million, crediting Ian Frazer's persistence for its decision. The Queensland government put its hand in its pocket too, with a cheque for $107 million, and he received strong support from Peter Beattie, after taking the former premier on a tour of a similar building overseas. With US philanthropist Chuck Feeney handing over a further $50 million, and smaller cheques being written by Queensland University of Technology and The University of Queensland, Ian moved into his new office in the $354 million Translational Research Institute building in 2012: a testament to his determination and business sense.

Ian's business acumen didn't just start and stop with what he could do inside the constraints of a university. He had set up his company Coridon and monitored how projects there were evolving, took on serious consultancies, including with Merck & Co., and joined with a couple of others to set up Implicit Bioscience, a bio-pharmaceutical company based in Brisbane and Seattle, which aims to develop drugs to modulate the human body's immune response to disease. Some of the work there is based on how the thymus gland works and centres around a compound that was discovered by the Russian military. Ian has invested in it too, backing its technology, providing a cash investment, becoming a foundation director, and continuing as chair of the company's scientific advisory board. Ian's interest is about three per cent, or $500,000, but mostly the company is made up of US angel investors. With involvement in those two companies – Coridon and Implicit Bioscience – Ian decided to finesse his business skills. Corporate governance and procedure worked very differently in the lab from around the boardroom table, so he enrolled in a night course a few years after Coridon was established in 2000, run by the Australian Institute of Company Directors.

Despite science being Ian's passion, it is his obsession with building 'the next big thing' that is the hallmark of his success. Along the way, that's meant a few casualties. While he's as generous as his schedule allows, the time he spends with his research students has progressively reduced, particularly during and since his tenure as 2006 Australian of the Year. So has the time he can spend on research. And he's had to rely on those key appointments on the way through, with his deputy, Ranjeny Thomas, picking up many of the pieces during his 2006 absences. Matt Brown has now taken over as head of the Diamantina Institute, which is part of the Translational Research Institute. With their three different personalities, together they have worked on a vision and created it.

Ian has been able to develop his strengths as his career has progressed: he's been the bench scientist, the administrator, the boss, the businessman, and the project manager. But in periods of introspection, he's also real about his faults. He tends to overcommit, leaving himself stretched, and sometimes disappointing those who need more of his time. That's not just Caroline and his family, but also some of his co-workers. And, as his senior team has learnt, he finds it hard to say no, and that's meant sometimes they've had to increase their workload, because he takes on too much. Caroline has spent forty years trying to open up the amount of time left for the family.

Early on, it was a combination of hard work but also the willingness to take a punt that paid off. Where many of his talented colleagues stayed in Edinburgh, he and Caroline tried their luck in Australia. When he could have made a career in Melbourne, he took the risk of moving again, to Brisbane. When his work on HIV was progressing well and earning good academic stripes, he decided to focus solely on HPV. Now, with his excess earnings going to philanthropic causes, he could go out on a high. But it's the lure of another cure, something else, that keeps him rising early, strapping on his cycling shoes, and riding to work. Ian Olver of Cancer Council Australia has no doubt there's another vaccine to come, saying Ian's HPV vaccine is just the first.

Ian's been helped by his ability not to lose sleep over anything anyone else might think. He just proceeds with absolute certainty that he's on the right path, whether it's driving in winter with the Peugeot roof down, playing loud music, or in the research laboratory. Bob Tindle remembers returning from a conference in Vancouver, where the Americans were talking about 'their' VLP invention, not acknowledging Ian or Jian in any way. He told Ian, who refused to be goaded into battle. Ian's view: who really cared? The fact remained that the discovery was made and a vaccine would result. The same attitude prevailed when a business deal soured between Ian and Mark Kendall, the biomedical engineer from Oxford who Ian had begun to mentor in business. Mark had planned to allow Coridon to license a technology he had developed, but then withdrew, believing his mojo was tied up with his intellectual property and it could be quickly swallowed up by the other work Coridon was doing. They continued to work together, and it was Ian, Mark says, who worked past the problems to dissolve any residual tensions. Mark is probably the person, apart from Caroline, who challenges Ian the most. The pair co-author grants and co-supervise students, but Mark remains in awe of the person who has given science a face in Australia.

What also helped Ian to grow from one job to the next was the level of independence he encouraged in his staff. He likes the people he works with, hates confrontation, and struggles to be tough with them. On one occasion, a colleague gave him a personal 'values' questionnaire to fill out, where the respondent had to prioritise their values – from integrity, to making a difference, to money – from five to one. The colleague remembers labouring over the questionnaire, but by the time she got back to her desk, Ian had already emailed through his answers. Spending time with friends at work headed his list: the enjoyment he got from the office was what he valued most. That's predominantly because of the like-mindedness he finds there. He relates to work, and to others with the same goals. This quality also became apparent to Peter Gray, the director of the Australian Institute for Bioengineering and Nanotechnology, when he lunched at Ian and Caroline's home in 2012. After a pear salad, where guests had to guess the dressing, a main course of fish, and Ian's signature lemon meringue pie, Peter thanked his hosts. 'That's fine,' Ian said. 'We'd all be working otherwise, wouldn't we?'

Ian's work at the Translational Research Institute will involve a new level of diplomacy. The board of directors, headed by David Watson, expects it to produce more as a group than the individual institutes would separately. Ian has to inspire the researchers there to believe that not only do they belong to their host university or institute, but that they also jointly belong to the new facility. This time it will be political, as much as strategic, as up to six hundred scientists work together on three major priorities: cancer (mainly skin, prostate and leukaemia), inflammation and autoimmunity, and diabetes. Inflammation is at the centre of the $350 million facility – as a driver of cancer, autoimmunity, and metabolic disorders like diabetes. The aim, which is the same around the world, is to better understand these diseases and build vaccines to get rid of them. The only respite Ian Frazer would enjoy in the early stages was to be atop a mountain, climbing out of a helicopter.

Nigel Spork was on his hands and knees. He could just make out his wife, Natasha, but visibility was almost zero and the noise deafening. The helicopter landed just a few metres away, using its big skids to settle on the snow. He was crunched down, watching the huge rotor blades do their work, with Natasha next to him and the couple that invited him along – Ian and Caroline Frazer – nearby. He couldn't see them, but they'd all gone through the same drill: keep your head down, stay put, beware of a rotor strike. They clambered onto the helicopter for the ride back down the mountain, the tenth and last of the day. Natasha, a Brisbane doctor, and Nigel, a businessman, loved skiing, but neither could remember a day of skiing quite so exhilarating. They were heli-skiing in Canada's Glacier National Park, and it was a holiday they would never forget.

It was Ian and Caroline's fourth heli-skiing holiday; the first one, in February 2010, got them both hooked, and this year they had returned with Nigel and Natasha, whom Ian had met at an entrepreneur of the year awards, and Brisbane medicos Bill and Linda Cockburn. The six of them were staying at Heather Mountain Lodge, just off the most northerly tip of the

Trans-Canada Highway in British Columbia's famous Rogers Pass. Like their other visits to Heather Mountain Lodge there were less than twenty-five guests at any one time, and that allowed daily use of the helicopter to ferry them up the virgin snow to the top of the mountain. By altitude standards, it wasn't very high, but it was snow that no one had stood on before, and it was a treat that only money could buy.

For years, Ian and Caroline had penny pinched to pay the mortgage, school their children, and, if enough existed at the end of the year, to take a modest holiday. Now, with royalties flowing in from the cervical cancer vaccine, their tastes hadn't changed. Big yachts held no appeal, nor a dozen houses. But skiing remained their number-one passion. Ian knew, for years, that he would have begged, borrowed or stolen to try this type of adventure holiday, but now he could afford it, and each year they would splurge for a week, with friends, high in the Canadian Rocky Mountains.

This holiday had been nutted out in detail over lunch at the Frazers' home. It was the first time Nigel and Natasha had met the Cockburns, but the six of them clicked immediately. Once in the snow though, talk was tough. Heli-skiing required focus, as well as fitness, and their days were packed with runs around trees, down the mountain and sometimes the odd fall. Deadly tree wells were disguised in the terrain: the snow settled on pine trees, covering them but leaving an air well, like the inside of a balloon, at its base. Skiers could topple headfirst into them; upside down, thick snow can fill your nose and mouth fast, and it's important to have someone nearby who can come to your aid. That's why heli-skiing involves a guide, who goes out in front, and a maximum of four skiers, in pairs. Experience doesn't help; luck dictates whether a tree well lies ahead. Natasha discovered this when she took a wrong turn one day and the guide was quick to rescue her. And Ian has been no stranger to the danger, having found himself trapped, upside down, several times.

There seemed to be no one else in the world, up there in the mountains, and ski lifts certainly weren't part of the scene. The snow was thick, almost impossible to walk in, and the unknown terrain meant they couldn't relax their focus. There were no places to stop for a coffee, and the powder snow made hard work of getting up after a fall. Small avalanches were not uncommon, and as the snow followed them downhill they all wondered how big the swell might become. They would have to ski out of it, or over it, a bit like surfing a wave.

At lunchtime, all the skiers would meet at a pre-designated spot. Seats were then carved out, cushions put on the ground, and the trusty choppers would arrive with eskies to deliver hot food and soup. Sweetened herbal tea was offered too, with Droste chocolates, providing energy for several more hours in the snow.

For Ian, it was also an escape from the computer. He loved his music and opera, but also enjoyed reading, particularly science fiction. As a child, he'd whipped through all the science fiction at the local library, seeing the plots more as instruction manuals than fantasy. And as time passed, he would pick up anything penned by Scottish author Iain Banks. He'd bookend his six hours' sleep each night with a book before going to bed, and his email within striking distance in the morning.

But it was the adventure that snow offers, along with the solitude of the slopes that had long appealed to Ian above other leisure pursuits. Without a natural flair for the team sports offered at school, he was quickly taken in by skiing. And with the ski runs around Aberdeen sometimes thin on snow, he soon graduated to the better snowfields across Europe. Skiing had also brought Ian and Caroline together, and it continued to be the sporting passion the couple shared, despite Caroline having smashed the top of her tibia into seventeen pieces on one trip to Whistler. Reaching speeds of one hundred kilometres per hour was fun, although Ian's risks were now calculated. His body wasn't as young as it was when he skied down a cliff face in Mürren, as a teenager, tied to his brother Ewan in the world's oldest ski race – the Scaramanga, in Switzerland.

Now, he tried to go to pilates with Caroline as much as he could. He felt fit, but flexibility was important too, and that was disappearing with the years. Cycling was his main exercise, but he didn't join the lycra brigade; it remained a necessary exercise, and it never offered the same joys he experienced atop a mountain of snow. Now, having discovered heli-skiing, he wouldn't wait until retirement to continue skiing. Each year, he vowed, he'd be back in the Canadian Rocky Mountains to catch a chopper up and down the slopes.

Other visiting Americans at the end of the table asked him what he did for a living. Nigel was listening for the answer. 'An academic,' Ian responded. Everyone was curious about each other. A joint like this didn't come cheaply, and intrigue followed the conversation around the table. The Americans persisted. What type of academic? 'A scientist,' he said. Nigel saw Caroline was smiling. Ian liked to be anonymous. That's why he loved dressing as Gene Simmons for the office Christmas party, hidden inside someone else's skin. That's why he loved leaving his mobile behind at the lodge each morning. That's why he wouldn't be mentioning to those holidaying with him that he needed to jump on a plane the next day, back to Australia, because he had been declared a national living treasure. And that's why there was no need to tell anyone who he was, or what he had done. He was certainly interested in having a good time though, and on the final evening an Italian group of skiers decided to get into the schnapps. Ian joined in, before singing an entire song – '*Am Schwarzen Walfisch*' – in German. On the way out, he and Caroline booked in for the next year.

Twenty-three

Between work and skiing, something else was marked regularly in Ian Frazer's diary, and today he was outside Woolworths at Indooroopilly shopping centre in Brisbane. He was sitting behind a table, with cakes piled high beside him. It was going to be a good morning, he knew it, as locals approached to purchase their annual Lions Club Christmas cake. The one-kilogram cakes sold for eleven dollars, and the 1.5-kilogram ones for fifteen dollars. Some of the shoppers had no idea who the tall Scotsman was; others had seen him before but couldn't figure out where it might have been. And then there were others who elbowed their friends in disbelief: 'Is that Ian Frazer, the famous scientist, selling Christmas cakes for charity?'

Ian, grateful for the funding help he received from the Lions Club when he moved to Brisbane in 1985, became an honorary member in the early 1990s. In the early 2000s, he became a regular at meetings and even took up the position of treasurer at his local branch. He liked the club's focus on health and the local community. He liked that members banded together to raise funds, decided together how to spend them, and that their activities ranged from sausage sizzles, to tree planting, to the annual Christmas cake drive.

His local branch, in Brisbane's inner west, gave away about twenty thousand dollars each year, and a big chunk of that – perhaps even as much as seventeen thousand dollars – came from selling cakes. Chris Simpson, the branch president, knew Ian helped sales; he was a drawcard, Chris says, and worked better than any big sign they could plaster around the place. The club booked this spot, just outside Woolies each year, from mid-November until Christmas Eve, and Ian would turn up to do his share of shifts. Chris remembers Ian arriving back from Europe on one occasion, with his body still in another time zone, and taking up the plastic chair at the charity table.

It was the same with branch meetings, on the first and third Tuesday of each month, in a roped-off area of the Indooroopilly Bowls Club. Ian just took his turn to speak, like everyone else. And he was committed. At a low point, the club was down to seven or eight members; and Ian and Caroline counted for two of those. Ian stayed out of any robust conversations, listened to what everyone said, sometimes checked his emails during long monologues, and would occasionally come in as the last person to offer a suggestion. People listened, Chris says. His priorities matched his wife's perfectly, and that was to first help those in their local community, whether they were needy families, single parents, or women's shelters. With each new project, Ian urged caution in choosing a recipient for their funds, and how donations would be granted. The Frazers believed in setting an example too, and that's why they took their turn barbecuing sausages and selling Christmas cakes. Ian didn't like the talk much; he liked rolling up his shirtsleeves and working. He was there to do a job.

Former branch president Ron Welsh was quick to see this, when Ian was elected as a fellow of The Royal Society in London. He sent Ian a congratulatory note, saying that he understood he might not be able to attend as many meetings. A response came back fast: evening work commitments were common, but Tuesdays were no better or worse than any other night, and he would continue to attend every Lions Club meeting that he could. And Ron was astonished at the next meeting, when Ian and Caroline Frazer walked through the door and took up their seats as usual.

Ian's parents, Sam and Marion Frazer, taught their children the importance of giving back, and it was a view shared strongly by Caroline. She and Ian never had much money in the early years, but they had each other, three healthy children, good friends, a strong education, and good jobs. If luck delivered you enough, it was important that you handed some on to others. Perhaps it was Ian's formative education, in Merchant Company schools, that had also imbued that philosophy. Early Edinburgh traders had 'salvaged their souls' by leaving money for education, and still today, schools in both Edinburgh and Aberdeen are supported by the Merchant Company. Or perhaps it was the Scottish ethic that meant you gave one-tenth of your wealth to charity; certainly in the Presbyterian Church that was expected, Ian, an atheist, would rather choose their beneficiaries; they could quickly write a cheque and save the time they give, but it defeated the purpose. To the Frazers, it was about service. Active involvement achieved much more long term, they believed, than any fat cheque might.

As the royalties for the vaccine flowed in, Ian and Caroline went from counting their pennies to wondering what to do with the excess. It ran into millions, and each year more flowed in.

With all the focus of a science experiment, they set about looking at priorities, and how they could ensure that any philanthropy they offered outlived them. The conversation kept coming back to two headline interests: education and the arts. They had both been gifted a good education and so had their children. They felt everyone deserved that. And the arts continued to be a passion, particularly opera, but also other music and a wide range of theatre. First up, they had to look after their three children. They didn't want to hand them a fortune but wanted to give them a leg-up. They decided the best option was property. If they had owned their own house earlier, they wouldn't have spent years paying off the mortgage and chasing their tails: they would have got ahead sooner. They paid their children's university fees and bought each of them an apartment, which they could sell, live in, or rent. From there, they had to find their own way, and the ongoing income would go to others.

In 2007, Ian and Caroline made an appointment to see their accountant. They adopted his sage advice immediately, setting up Frazer Services Pty Ltd as trustee for the Frazer Family Trust, along with the Frazer Family Foundation. The foundation would be a private auxiliary fund, receiving donations from Ian and Caroline Frazer and then distributing them to charities. Even before the money came rolling in, they had given small amounts to particular causes, and they wanted to keep that up. The Leukaemia Foundation was one of those.

Caroline, while teaching in Brisbane, saw three children die of the disease. And the tragic circumstances around each of those deaths had stayed with her. One little boy was diagnosed in year three; he had a sister who stood by while their parents did everything they possibly could. He was in and out of school, in and out of remission, and then lost his life in his first year of high school. A second little girl was diagnosed in preschool and lost her life the next year. A third child was diagnosed in year five, surviving for two years. That kind of wretchedness stays with a school, and each year Caroline would write a small cheque with those three families in the forefront of her mind. Now, it went down on her list: she wanted to ensure the Leukaemia Foundation received a donation from the Frazer Family Foundation.

And so the pair nutted out how they could annually support a list of charities with which they felt connected: the Cancer Council Queensland, which had supported Ian before he became a household name, Smiling for Smiddy, which combined the need to raise funds for cancer with Ian's love of cycling, and even Surf Life Saving Australia, once their son Callum joined the beach brigade. Support for The University of Queensland Immunotherapy Research Travel Fund was crucial to ensure that young scientists were able to keep up with international best practice, National Parks Queensland, and the Princess Alexandra Research Foundation, where Ian sat as a board member, all featured on their list. It was not a plan to pay back the help the Frazers had received along the way; it stemmed from the simple belief that if you have more than enough, it should be shared around. The one million dollar donation, earmarked to provide cervical cancer vaccines for schoolgirls in Vanuatu, was also set aside.

Education bound the Frazer family. All of their children were high achievers at school, and both Caroline, who did her master's with three young children under her feet, and Ian believed it opened doors to opportunities that everyone should be afforded. Ian knew that his grants were funded each year by the public purse, allowing him to do his research. Australia doesn't have the tradition of supporting universities in the same way Americans support colleges in the United States, but Ian was determined to set an example. When a campaign to encourage University of Queensland staff to donate back to the university through their pay packets began, Ian thought it was useless for the people at the top to ask others to donate if they weren't doing the same themselves. So he put one hundred thousand dollars on the table, saying it was there on the basis that each year it was matched by staff. There is a rider: it will remain as long as public funding, via federal grants, continues for those employed in his laboratory. He wasn't going to have his staff working around the clock to have their jobs cut for political expediency. If he had to, he says, he'd pay them himself.

Certainly, he's done that before. When one senior staff member's grant wasn't renewed, he ensured he kept his job, with a research assistant. The one million dollars he was awarded as the Balzan Prize winner went straight back into the work money pot. So too did the three hundred thousand dollars given to him in 2008 for the Prime Minister's Science Prize. The prize money should be gifted back to scientific research, Ian thought, because it had been awarded for research.

Tamino, the handsome prince in Mozart's opera *The Magic Flute*, is being chased by a serpent. He collapses and three young women, attendants of the Queen of the Night, appear and kill the serpent. Each wants the prince for herself, and with no compromise, they all leave. Tamino recovers to hear the bird catcher Papageno take credit for killing the serpent. The three young ladies reappear and punish him. They show Tamino a portrait of a beautiful young woman called Pamina. He falls in love on the spot. Pamina's mother then enters the stage, played on this occasion by twenty-something Brisbane-based soprano Milica Ilic. She tells Tamino that her daughter has been captured by her enemy and demands he rescue her, promising that he can marry her daughter in return.

Milica, they say in opera circles, has a big future ahead, helped along by the tens of thousands of dollars Ian and Caroline gift to Opera Queensland each year. The money, which is assigned to the young artists' program, helps pay for voice, movement, and language coaches, which many students could not afford otherwise. Milica is certainly one of them. Born in Serbia, before living in New Zealand and then Brisbane, she trained at the Queensland Conservatorium. But it was the added help given to her by Ian and Caroline's personal patronage in 2010 that has given her performances what she calls a 'trampolining effect'. Ian has also spoken to her, as he does others he personally supports at both Opera Queensland and the Queensland Symphony Orchestra, inquiring about her goals and inspirations. He especially likes supporting sopranos, and is specific about the money being used to develop the talent they are already showing. A symmetry exists in his mind between art and science: young scientists scrimp and save to win regular grants to etch out a career, and young artists are no different.

Opera Queensland's artistic director Lindy Hume found out, when she took the couple to dinner in late 2012, how much Ian knows about opera. Not only was he specific about advancing young talent with the couple's donations, but he passionately launched into robust conversations about everything from characters, to different roles, to the direction of the company. He will do the same with those from the Queensland Symphony Orchestra, or in chats about Musica Viva. It's not a knowledge built up overnight: he and Caroline don't have to sit in the cheap seats any more, like they did at university, and now they have access to money, it is even more reason to provide big chunks of it to Queensland's arts scene. But opera, especially, holds a special place, with its entertainment, theatre, and music all rolled into one. They never tire of it, and Mozart's *The Magic Flute*, which Ian thinks shows Mozart at his best, probably tops the list; he has seen it almost twenty times. Puccini's *Tosca* is also high on his favourites' list. He loves the melodrama, set in 1800, with the Kingdom of Naples' control of Rome threatened by Napoleon's invasion of Italy. It's a 'community rebellion of repressive governments'-type story, which Ian finds especially appealing.

Caroline and Ian's relationship is not a complex one: they've worked together as a team – whether cleaning up after a dinner party, planning a family holiday, or fundraising – since marrying almost forty years ago. A common set of values has helped, and a sense of pragmatism, where the value of money is in the advantage it offers. But there are just as many differences as similarities, particularly when it comes to personality. Ian is reserved, even shy. He doesn't seek the limelight, but has learnt that it can help achieve an end. The exterior portrayal of certainty that beams out from the television hides the same self-doubts the rest of us have. It's just that he doesn't look for affirmation. He's Ian. Caroline is more social, emotional, and gregarious, and her ability to talk to anyone has helped Ian along the way. If Ian's stressed, he might misplace his tie. She will know where it is immediately. If she's upset, he knows what to say to soothe her. It works for them both.

Within months of arriving in Australia, they had a newborn and no local family support, and they learnt to depend on each other one hundred per cent. Caroline has made the lion's share of sacrifices, but Ian's absences have become easier as technology has improved. Now, when he goes away, they can talk daily – unlike the long trips when the children were still small. Once, Ian would sit under the stairs at his desk at home, because that was where the computer was housed. Now he's on the sofa at the end of a long day, reading an electronic document. Caroline will sit next to him, watching a movie or reading a book. Little strategies like this have helped their union. So has Caroline's determination to always make times in their diary for the two of them; she knows that if she doesn't get in first, the dates will be swallowed by Ian's work. Pilates, when Ian's in town, is something they enjoy together. So too is the work they do with the Lions Club, and the skiing trips they can now afford when they like. The same goes for opera.

The Frazers don't put their wealth on public display. They don't flaunt it, and that means they can be glaring omissions from rich lists and charity hunters. The Frazer Foundation is one of more than eight hundred philanthropic foundations across Australia and flies under the radar. Caroline especially likes that, thinking it's better to keep their arts donations private. But Ian sees that differently, particularly when it comes to the arts. 'You have to lead by example,' he told her, and that means being public about their patronage. It's the same type of thinking behind his gift-matching scheme at The University of Queensland. So Ian and Caroline are public about a couple of donations, even appealing to others to join them in a philanthropic bid to keep the arts strong in their home state. *Opera companies can only offer opera if they have the necessary resources* – the couple wrote in a message to other potential donors – *talented people, both on the stage and behind the stage, and access to the costumes, stage sets and music that makes opera special. That's where we and you can help. We wanted to ensure that there would continue to be opera in Queensland and produced by Queenslanders for Queenslanders.*

It mirrors Ian's thinking in Lions Club conversations too. Charity begins at home, and you must look at helping your own local communities; in this case the local arts community. With the exception of Vanuatu, and the need for the vaccine to be accessed in developing countries, the Frazers' charity recipients are grassroots organisations where no money is chewed up in administrative fees. *We decided some years ago to give a regular donation to help Opera Queensland with their work,* Ian and Caroline's message continues. *We're now asking you to consider doing the same.*

It's a strong public advertisement, similar to putting Ian on a plastic chair outside Woolies to sell Christmas cakes, or on billboards across the city in a bid to boost enrolments at The University of Queensland. And it's worth at least as much again as the couple gives personally.

Twenty-four

The year twelve students at Springfield College on Brisbane's outskirts pour through the doors and take a seat in front of Leisa Ashton from the Australian Cervical Cancer Foundation. It's cold, winter 2012, but their focus is firmly on the young woman standing in front of them. Four in every five students in the room, she says, will come in contact with HPV some time in their lifetime. HPV. Does anyone know what it is?

Leisa looks around the room. She has done this many times before, at many schools. And Springfield College is no different from other high schools she has visited. All the female students have received the vaccine against HPV, but it's clear as soon as she asks the questions that they haven't really understood why. HPV is a virus spread through sexual contact, Leisa tells them: 'It's the common cold of being sexually active.' The students stifle giggles, the males in the room wondering why they've been invited along with their female classmates. Some of them keep their eyes cast down, and Leisa answers the question they are asking themselves. It's as big an issue for boys as it is for girls, she says, because ten per cent of people who die from an HPV-related cancer are male. Those cancers include anal, penile, and throat cancers. They should all remember too, she says, that they have mothers and sisters.

Then Jade Goody, the young outspoken woman from the Big Brother series in the United Kingdom, hits the screen. She's bigger and louder than life on the screen, but these teenagers also know that Jade died of cervical cancer in 2009, on Mother's Day. She was just a decade older than some of them now, aged twenty-seven. The students look at the wedding videos of Jade, in the throes of dying, which now fill the screen in front of the room. The room is silent. The boys who had their eyes cast down are now staring at the video. So are the girls. Jade Goody was like them. She was young and brash and seemingly immortal. And now she is dead, courtesy of cervical cancer. The film fades and Leisa knows she has this group in the palm of her hand.

She sees their faces, their awkward uneasiness, and turns a negative into a plus. Cervical cancer is the only cancer that can be prevented by a vaccine, she says, because it makes the body produce its own immunity against the cancer-causing HPV strains. Forty million women have now been given the vaccine, from the doctors' surgeries of Brisbane to those in Latvia, from New York City to Romania, South Korea, Slovenia, and dozens of other countries. It's saving lives every day, she says, people like their sisters and mothers. And young, confident people like Jade Goody too.

Leisa ends the session with the students fighting over quiz prizes. What is HPV? How many people will contract it in their lifetime? Hands shoot up all over the place. Boys and girls. She gives out a few prizes, ensuring that none of the boys wins a make-up kit, and packs up knowing the session has been successful.

She doesn't know yet that Australia, within weeks, will become the first country to also vaccinate boys, with the vaccine rolled out to twelve- and thirteen-year-olds nationally. That twenty-million dollar four-year program, which was announced in July 2012, will protect boys from genital warts, some cancers, and also stop HPV being passed onto women who haven't been vaccinated. It is estimated that one-quarter of new infections will be avoided by extending the vaccine to boys.

Already Ian Frazer's vaccine was making a stunning dent in the number of deaths that occurred each year from cervical cancer. According to experts, the rates of genital warts has dropped by ninety per cent in young women, and eighty per cent in young men, an early indicator that cervical cancer can fall by similar amounts. Of course, the vaccine must also be distributed in developing countries, where mortality rates are the highest.

This is the point that occupies Ian Frazer's mind. It's not just about logistics, it's also a fight against poverty, with billions needed to ensure every woman can access the vaccine, and ignorance, with women even in Australia still unaware that HPV is the most likely cause of cervical cancer. It is two steps forward, one step back, and that's the dance that science has demanded since Ian Frazer started. This and that works, so you take two steps forward. This doesn't, so you go back a step to work out why. Something unexpected works sometimes, which is akin to a shuffle to the side.

Science has given Ian the ride of a lifetime. The public acknowledgement he can take or leave, and the same goes for the riches that have come with it. But he's appreciated the opportunity to travel the world – from holding a panda cub on his knee in China, to celebrating his recent sixtieth birthday in

Antarctica, to sleeping out in the Sossusvlei Desert in Namibia, to visiting the royal palace in Bhutan. Caroline, on each trip, pinches herself; she remembers those long years when every cent was saved in the hope of having a small family holiday. Now she counts an unlikely snow shower in Uluru, their regular Canadian heli-skiing trips, and a dance performance in an intimate theatre in St Petersburg as her holiday highlights. And Turtle Island in Fiji, closer to home, has a special lure for Caroline, because it impedes Ian's ability to work. The couple bid for – and won – a holiday to the island at a charity auction to raise money for cancer research. The fact that it didn't have mobile phone reception, and its one computer was housed in the resort office – offering internet speed akin to dial-up – particularly impressed Caroline. She'll continue her bid for a bigger chunk of Ian's time, as he savours the opportunity to keep on building – whether it's a vaccine to save lives, a new facility that integrates science and medicine, or the knowledge base of students.

Ian's in front of his own class now, and it's not at Springfield College. He's in a room at the Princess Alexandra Hospital with his students, explaining that something needs to be retested. This is a regular part of his week, hearing where his students are up to, and offering advice on what the next step might be. Building their knowledge. First up today is Le Son Tran, a PhD student. He takes to the lectern, with Ian Frazer in the front row. Ian's other postdoctoral students, research assistants, and team leaders – who make up the Frazer Lab – are sitting, listening, too. Some of them have brought their own lunch, but a steady flow of cake makes its way around the room. Le Son Tran has been dealing with mice, grafting the ear skin of one that expresses HPV proteins onto an immunocompetent, syngeneic mouse. The aim is to see if the recipient mouse recognises the viral protein and is able to reject it. Son has been working on the problem for ages, as part of his PhD, and there have been ups and downs. He doesn't like the downs; he wants affirmation that the experiment he is conducting is working. He did his bachelor's and master's in Vietnam and arrived in Australia as an international student after finding Ian Frazer's name on the internet. He wrote him a letter and Ian emailed back, asking him to apply for a scholarship, which he did. Now he works six days a week, and you can see he wants to impress his boss in the front row.

Son says it's Ian's way of thinking that has captivated him. When Son did his initial experiment, the mouse didn't reject the graft, showing that the HPV could evade the normal immune system. That wasn't what Son was expecting, and he admits to feeling discouraged. Ian taught him how to turn a negative into a positive, Son says. He now knows that a negative finding means you can rule something out, which refines your next step. Ian has also affected *how* Son works. Good scientists, Son explains, don't do research work one hundred per cent of the time, only two-thirds of the time. The remainder should be spent thinking and reading, and that's what he plans to pass on to his students, eventually, when he realises his dream of returning to Vietnam and lecturing in science.

But right now, Son is front and centre. He talks about things most of us have never heard of – from arginase-1 mediating DNCB-induced inflammation, to the effect of arginase inhibitor on the ear swelling of mice. Ian jots down a few notes, not many, but enough to prompt him when Son has completed his presentation. Ian asks several questions: they are always polite but don't miss their mark. 'If someone disagrees with me, say so,' Ian Frazer says. No one does.

The Tuesday presentations are locked in Ian's diary; it's how he catches up with what is happening in his lab, and his students receive the feedback they need. Son now knows what he will focus on next. Today's presentations will be shorter than usual, curtailed slightly because – as Ian explains to his students – US billionaire Chuck Feeney is in town and has agreed to see him. 'And that's an appointment I don't want to miss,' he says. But the presentations will continue at the same time next week, because, like benchwork, Ian divides the week up. Some days are given over to administration and oversight of the Translational Research Institute; and others revolve around the laboratory work he is listening to now – which could hold the key to so much more.

It's a delicate balancing act, now he's at the helm of the big, new facility. His diary fills with board meetings, strategy meetings and finance meetings. Meetings are held over fire safety, and whether sheds can be moved from one place to another. The meeting that follows the one on fire safety might have Ian, with his hand out, asking for research dollars. And then the health minister wants to see him, along with the chief operating officer, and the financial controller. He's an administrator these days, more than a scientist, and he knows it. He hasn't done any serious benchwork for a decade, and that's why he likes the days when he's back nearer the bench, closer to the mice, and what they might be hiding.

So what's the next step for Ian Frazer? On some days he says it could be retirement atop a snow-covered mountain, with no phone and only Caroline at his side. He's got the money to do that. But it's hard to imagine. He admits that retirement moment might be a long way away. He knows that the next question might just lead to the therapeutic vaccine to cure those women already fighting cervical cancer. Or the next step might herald the vaccine he's working on for herpes, or for skin cancer. There's more to build. It's always the thought of the next step that drives Ian Hector Frazer.

Ian's Lemon meringue pie

Ingredients

Pastry
70 g self-raising flour
130 g plain flour
30 g caster sugar
120 g cold butter, chopped
1 large egg

Meringue
3 large egg whites
170 g caster sugar

Lemon filling
60 g cornflour
170 g sugar
180 ml fresh lemon juice
230 ml water
60 g butter, chopped
3 large egg yolks

Method

1. To make the pastry, place the self-raising and plain flours, caster sugar, and butter in a food processor. Process on medium speed for about 20 seconds, or until the mixture resembles fine breadcrumbs (there shouldn't be any large chunks of butter). Add the egg and continue to process on medium speed for about 15–30 seconds, or until the egg is incorporated and the mixture clumps together.

2. Form the dough into a flattened disc and place in a freezer bag or wrap in plastic wrap. Refrigerate for at least 1 hour.

3. To make the lemon filling, combine the cornflour, sugar, lemon juice and water in a saucepan. Stir until the mixture is smooth. Place over medium–high heat and stir constantly until the mixture starts to boil (this will probably take about 7–10 minutes). Reduce the heat to low and continue stirring for about 30–40 seconds, or until the mixture changes from cloudy to transparent and becomes thick and smooth. Remove from the heat and vigorously stir in the butter and egg yolks. Continue stirring until all the butter has melted and the ingredients are well combined. Pour the lemon filling into a small container, cover, and refrigerate until cold.

4. Preheat the oven to 180°C (160°C fan-forced). If you are not using a fan-forced oven, adjust the oven rack to the lower middle position. Lightly grease a 23 cm round pie dish.

5. Roll out the pastry between two sheets of baking paper to make a circle with a 29 cm diameter, about 4 mm thick. Gently press into the dish to line the base and side and trim any overhanging pastry. Place a sheet of baking paper on top of the pastry and fill with pastry weights or uncooked rice. Bake for 10 minutes, then remove the weights and baking paper and bake for 10–15 minutes further, until the pastry is a light, golden colour. Allow the pastry shell to cool completely.

6. Increase the oven temperature to 200°C (190°C fan-forced). If you are not using a fan-forced oven, adjust the oven rack to the middle position.

7. To make the meringue, place the egg white in the bowl of an electric mixer and beat on high speed until at soft peak

stage (when the beater is lifted, a peak will form and then droop over). Add the sugar gradually, about 2 tablespoons at a time, beating well after each addition. Once all the sugar has been added, continue beating until the sugar has dissolved and the mixture is thick and glossy. To test whether the sugar has dissolved, rub a small amount of meringue between your thumb and finger. If you can still feel sugar crystals, beat the meringue for another minute, then test again.

8. Spoon the lemon filling into the cooled pastry shell and spread evenly. Dollop the meringue on top of the lemon filling, then spread the meringue to cover the filling. Form peaks in the meringue with a spoon (press the back of a spoon against the surface of the meringue, then lift the spoon to form a peak).

9. Bake for about 7–10 minutes, or until the meringue is lightly coloured. Allow the pie to cool to room temperature, then cover and refrigerate until cold. Slice the chilled pie into wedges and serve.

Recipe published courtesy of
www.exclusivelyfood.com.au

ACKNOWLEDGEMENTS

To write someone's biography requires an extraordinary openness and honesty on behalf of the subject. Ian Frazer provided that in spades, along with good humour and enormous patience in explaining the science behind his work. Thank you Ian. Life is enriched by those you meet – I will treasure the time we spent together for years to come. Ian's generosity of time and spirit was probably only matched by that of his wife, Caroline. Caroline's hospitality, willingness to open up family albums, and help in getting me inside the head of her husband was crucial. Indeed, without Caroline's support it's doubtful whether Ian would have reached such lofty heights; nor would this book be published. Xiao Yi Sun will be a friend for life. Even though the death of her brilliant husband Jian is still raw, she opened up to me, ensuring both Ian's and Jian's place in history is recorded

So many other people helped build a picture of Ian – thank you to his parents, Marion and Sam, his three children, his brothers and their families. To his childhood friends, who now marvel that the tall skinny lad from next door rose to become

Australian of the Year, thanks for taking the calls in the middle of the night, and delving into past decades to bring Ian's childhood alive. The same appreciation goes to school friends, university colleagues, teachers, and tutors who clearly remember the student who stood out in Aberdeen, Edinburgh and Melbourne many years ago. Ian Mackay was especially helpful.

To the staff at the Walter and Eliza Hall Institute, past and present, your willingness to check facts and open doors has been genuinely appreciated. The same goes for the team at CSL, particularly John Cox and Peter Turvey, who were crucial for my understanding of patent issues. John, I owe you more than a bottle of red! Professor Jeff Dunn and his colleagues taught me important funding and research issues and dozens of Ian's colleagues filled in gaps along the way. To Joe Tooma, Leisa Ashton and the crew at ACCF, thanks for your unbridled enthusiasm and hard work in spreading the message about cervical cancer.

Family and friends often feature in acknowledgements, but I want to particularly thank Robert King for his pedantic proofreading, Dr Brigid Hickey who reads more books than anyone I know, Jamie Walker for his professional insights, and my husband David Fagan whose encouragement is limitless. To Sue Carson, Margaret Dwyer, Dr Amanda McKee, Ardena Ulliana and Chrissi Stanicic, you can start inviting me places again.

The idea for this book came from UQP publisher Madonna Duffy, whose inspiration, determination, kind words and thoughtful approach made it a pleasure. The team effort at UQP makes you want to have books published there. Rebecca Roberts' editing skills were matched only by her determination not to give birth to her first child before deadline. Thanks Rebecca. And to Jacqueline Blanchard, who took over, thank you for asking all those questions that needed to be answered.

Index